Making Change Work for You in Health Care

by Richard S. Deems. Ph.D.,
and K. C. Warner, R.Ph.

American Media Incorporated
4900 University Avenue
West Des Moines, IA 50266-6769
800-262-2557
ami@ammedia.com

Making Change Work for You in Health Care

Richard S. Deems, Ph.D., and K. C. Warner, R.Ph.
Copyright © 1998 by American Media Inc.

All rights reserved. No part of this publication may be reproduced, stored in a retrieval system, or transmitted, in any form or by any means, electronic, mechanical, photocopying, recording, or otherwise, without the prior written permission of the publisher.

This publication is designed to provide accurate and authoritative information in regard to the subject matter covered. It is sold with the understanding that neither the author nor the publisher is engaged in rendering legal, accounting, or other professional service. If legal advice or other expert assistance is required, the services of a competent professional should be sought.

Credits:
American Media Publishing: Art Bauer
                              Todd McDonald
Managing Editor: Karen Massetti Miller
Designer: Gayle O'Brien

Published by American Media Inc.
4900 University Avenue
West Des Moines, IA 50266-6769

Library of Congress Catalog Card Number 98-70378
Deems, Richard S., Ph.D., and Warner, K. C., R.Ph.
Making Change Work for You in Health Care

Printed in the United States of America
1998
ISBN 1-884926-85-1

Acknowledgments

Over the years, many people have contributed to this work, including the participants in our workshops and training sessions. CEO Larry Pugh and managers and leaders at Allen Memorial Hospital energetically added their insights on ways to deal with change, as did key leaders from IASD Health Services Corp.

Kathy Kolbe and her books *The Conative Connection: Uncovering the Link Between Who You Are and How You Perform* (Addison Wesley, 1990) and *Pure Instinct; Business' Untapped Resource* (Time Books/Random House, 1993) have given us significant insight into how people differ in the ways they naturally respond to change. We would also like to thank Dr. Roger Hiemstra, an expert in adult learning; the cotrainers who have worked with us over the years; Todd McDonald, who kept us honest and logical in the way we presented this information; Karen Massetti Miller, for her editorial work; Art Bauer, who consistently conveyed confidence in our work; physicians Elwood Yaw, Kennedy Fawcett, and Larry Gray; insurance executive Chuck Rohm; and Sandie Deems.

Additional thanks go to the talented colleagues who have provided us with invaluable insights into the health-care industry: Kathy Berdusco, R.Ph., Searle Pharmaceutical; Elizabeth McCullough, Hospice; Gary Butkus, R.Ph., Searle Pharmaceutical; Charles Cannon, M.D., Enid Gastroenterology; Larry Cannon; Shari Cannon, Blackwell Regional Hospital; Tom Cannon; Laura K. Davis; Pam Fronberger, Premier, Inc.; Rhonda Haggard, R.Ph., Medi-Save; Andy Harnett, AstraMerck Inc.; Elaine Ketner, VHA; Karen Lawson, Ph.D.; John Phillips, R.Ph., Eli Lilly & Company; Cathy Swindell, R.Ph., Walgreen's Pharmacy; Paula Snyder, St. Vincent Hospital System; Ken Weidner, University of Chicago Hospital; and Michael Williams, Glaxo Wellcome.

Introduction

If you work in health care and are going through some kind of organizational change—or if you have gone through a major change and now want to make sense of it all—then you are not alone. This book will help you understand yourself and other health-care professionals and the dynamics of the change process within health care. Our goal is to provide you with the information you need to become your own expert at making change work for you—whether it's organizational change or personal change.

Although people don't always welcome change, change is usually a positive force in our lives. At least that's been the experience of the authors. As we look back at our personal and professional lives, we realize that when there hasn't been enough change, we created it.

Richard S. Deems traces his interest in the subject of change back to high school and to his fascination with books that described what happens to people and organizations in change, including Alvin Toffler's *Future Shock* and Lyle E. Schaller's *Understanding Tomorrow*. In college and as part of his graduate studies, Richard took courses dealing with the topic of change; his doctoral research focused on what happens to people who go through the experience of moving from one community to another. Later while going through the experience of being fired, he devoted a lot of personal energy analyzing his own reactions to the process of change.

As a health-care provider, K. C. Warner was intrigued by the changes that occurred in her field during the past decade. She found that patients and providers were approaching the caregiving process differently than they had in the past. Both K. C and Richard want to meet the challenge of working through health-care change to provide the best patient care possible.

As we consider this challenge, it seems that, contrary to what we have read in certain books, change in health care is not a neat, linear, sequential kind of process that moves from endings to new beginnings. It's much more dynamic, more fluid, more interactive, more up and down. If it were an amusement park ride, it would be more like a roller coaster than a merry-go-round; if it were a shape, it would be more free-form than rectangular.

Since we first began studying change, we've worked with several thousand people who've experienced it firsthand, especially in the unique health-care setting. They've made invaluable contributions to this book by sharing their insights and providing feedback on the interactive exercises. You'll read about the success strategies many of them used to deal with change in their own lives. We hope that you are able to use the information in this book to become your own expert at making change work for you in the exciting, dynamic world of health care.

Richard S. Deems, Ph.D., and K. C. Warner, R.Ph.

How to Read This Book

This book has been designed to be as user friendly as possible. The writing style is easy to understand, and the organization is easy to follow. The interactive exercises included are designed to help you think through the information so you can apply it to your situation right away.

Here are several suggestions to help you get the most from *Making Change Work for You in Health Care:*

- First take a few minutes to flip through the book, letting your eyes fall on whatever headings or paragraphs grab your attention and reading whatever interests you. Get acquainted with the book and how it's organized. Read the authors' comments in the Introduction.

- Next turn to the Table of Contents and look at the chapter titles and major topics. As you read the chapter titles, ask yourself, "What chapters seem to address the same questions I have about how to make change work in health care?" and "What other questions do I have about making change work in health care?" Make a list of all your questions.

- Then begin reading Chapter 1, "Identifying Change in Health Care." Be honest in your own assessment of what you are experiencing in your health-care setting.

- Continue reading the book. The next chapters will explore the situations that are bringing you here in the first place. They'll look into how much you already know about change and change in health care, and how people naturally vary in their reactions to change. Later chapters will give you the strategies you need to make change work for you, including tips on managing the stress that often accompanies change. The last chapter will help you design your own Plan for Action to make change work in health care.

After you've read the book from cover to cover, you may want to return to the sections you found most helpful to reinforce the points they make. Here are some tips to help you:

- Take a sheet of paper and write out three questions you still have about change in health care. In your first question, identify a key word or phrase that might indicate where in the book you'll find the answer.

- Return to the Table of Contents and skim the chapter titles and major topics to identify the areas where you might find the answer. Reread the material in those sections until your question has been answered.

- Repeat this procedure for the rest of your questions. As you find answers to each of them, you may come up with still other questions. If you do, just continue the process.

The publisher and authors hope you find this book insightful and helpful and that it will be one you frequently pull off the shelf to revisit. Our goal is to help you become your own expert at making change work for you in health care.

Table of Contents

Chapter 1

Identifying Change in Health Care — 10

Managing Wellness — 11
Partnering with Patients — 12
Working with New Technologies — 12
Working in Changing Treatment and Recovery Settings — 13
Adapting to New Ownership and New Structures — 13

Chapter 2

What We Already Know About Change — 16

Dynamic 1: Self-Chosen Change Is the Easiest — 17
Dynamic 2: We Are What We Are Because of Change — 18
Dynamic 3: The Way Work Gets Done Is Rapidly Changing — 19
Dynamic 4: Change That Affects Relationships Is the Most Difficult — 22
Dynamic 5: Change Is Constant — 23

Chapter 3

Why Everyone Doesn't React to Change the Same Way — 24

Conation: How We Naturally Get Things Done — 25
The Kolbe Conative Action Modes™ — 25
Conative Strengths and Organizational Change — 33

Chapter 4

Guiding Your Team's Reaction to Change — 36

Setting the Stage: Rumors and the Announcement — 37
Stage 1: Positioning — 37
Stage 2: Uncertainty — 39
Stage 3: Clarification — 40
Stage 4: Focus — 41
Stage 5: Acceptance — 41
Resistance and Exit — 42
Guiding Your Team's Reaction — 43

Chapter 5
Managing Stress Effectively — 46

    Strategy 1: Use Your Endorphins — 47
    Strategy 2: Talk It Out — 49
    Strategy 3: Anticipate Times of Stress — 49
    Strategy 4: Reward Yourself — 50
    Strategy 5: Volunteer — 51
    Strategy 6: Go for a Drive — 51
    Strategy 7: Use Moderation — 51
    Strategy 8: Use Your Conative Strengths — 52
    Strategy 9: Interact with a Pet — 54
    Strategy 10: Challenge Your Mind-Set — 54
    Still More Strategies — 55

Chapter 6
Seven Strategies for Making Change Work in Health Care — 58

    Strategy 1: View Change As Opportunity — 59
    Strategy 2: Be Someone Others Enjoy Working With — 60
    Strategy 3: Practice Effective Stress-Management Strategies — 61
    Strategy 4: Build Bridges, Not Fences — 62
    Strategy 5: Exit If You Must — 64
    Strategy 6: Ask the Consultant's Question — 65
    Strategy 7: Know What You Do Best and Where You Best Fit — 68

Chapter 7
Dealing with Downsizings — 72

    Take Action to Stay in Control — 72
    Following the Deems Job Loss Reaction Cycle™ — 75

Chapter 8
Developing a Plan for Action — 80

    Identify Your Questions — 80
    Develop Strategies for Turning Plans into Reality — 84
    Create Your Plan for Action — 90

Chapter One

Identifying Change in Health Care

Do you ever wonder what will happen next in health care? What will the next organizational or technological change be? What new processes or procedures will it create? And, perhaps most importantly, how can you work successfully with change once it occurs?

If you want to deal effectively with organizational change in health care, you need to know how to make change work for you. This book will help you do just that. But be prepared—making change work requires more than just reading a few pages or talking about change with your team. To make change work for you, you'll need to think about what you read and reflect on your discussions. You'll also need to take action by:

- Identifying the changes taking place in your organization.
- Committing yourself to making that change work for you.
- Mastering the skills that will make you your own change expert.

> **Change is all around us; in fact, it's the norm in today's health-care organizations.**

Change is all around us; in fact, it's the norm in today's health-care organizations. The fact that one industry can manage through so much change in such a short amount of time is amazing. Insurance plans change. Patients change. Technologies change. Staff members change. Procedures change.

Not too long ago, health care was represented by the TV persona of Marcus Welby, M.D. When a patient felt ill, that person visited the family doctor, paid for the visit, picked up a prescription, went home, and got better. Now health care is considered an industry. Workflow has changed for the caregiver, and the patient's experience with providers has changed too.

The pace of change in health care today is so rapid that we can't outline everything that is happening. Besides, most of these changes have a cause-and-effect action—each change sets in motion other, future changes that are not always identifiable at the moment. However, after listening to thousands of health-care employees and considering the entire health-care industry, we can point to several emerging trends that have had, or will have, a direct impact on everyone involved in providing health-care services:

- Managing wellness
- Partnering with patients
- Working with new technologies
- Working in changing treatment and recovery settings
- Adapting to new ownership and new structures

Managing Wellness

One of the most significant changes in health care is the shifting emphasis from taking care of the sick to preventing illness and managing wellness. This is a major movement toward prevention rather than cure, preventing illness and disease rather than just easing pain or curing an illness or injury after it's occurred. This affects both health-care providers and health-care customers, and it calls for a shift in mind-set.

> **Instead of working with the sick, health-care providers will increasingly work with those who are well and want to stay that way.**

Instead of working with the sick, health-care providers will increasingly work with those who are well and want to stay that way. Though we will still need trauma centers and intensive care units, more and more health-care professionals will shift their emphasis to coaching patients in how to prevent illness.

What drives this shift to managing wellness? Some say it's the natural extension of the earlier wellness movement that pushed for smoke-free work environments, in-house fitness facilities, and other actions to help keep people healthy. Others say the push to managing wellness is merely economical. It costs less to prevent illness than to treat it. Others say it is an extension of education—people know more about health and are willing to spend time and money to prevent illness rather than cure it.

Whether it's an economic issue or a values issue has little impact on the bottom line: health-care providers' work is shifting from curing the sick to managing wellness.

Identifying Change in Health Care

Partnering with Patients

Patients are changing. We know this, but sometimes we forget the way it impacts our care. One way patients are changing is that they are becoming more consumer focused. For example, research shows that patients leaving a health-care institution report that they are more concerned about how they were treated than getting well. Patients are becoming more educated, more aware of differences in care, and ready to compare the care from various providers.

Social gatherings often include at least one conversation about how well or not-so-well a person was treated by a doctor or local hospital. Patients are starting to shop for health-care services.

The look of the patient population is changing also. The surge of population labeled "baby boomers" is approaching early retirement age. As the boomers continue to age, they will place additional pressure on the health-care system. The sheer number of people who are retired or of retirement age will have an impact on health care.

> **Patients are taking more control of their own care.**

Perhaps the most significant change, however, is that patients are taking more control of their own care. Historically, patients felt that the doctor, pharmacist, or nurse knew what was best for them and seldom questioned their care. They would "follow the doctor's orders." Increasingly patients want to be involved in managing their own health and be part of the health-care team.

Today's patient wants to know why—why one medication is recommended over another, why one procedure is used rather than an alternative, and on what basis the diagnosis and prognosis have been made. Increasingly patients are researching their health conditions and treatment options and wanting to be involved in the management of their own care. Name any illness, and you can find a great deal of information somewhere on the Internet.

Partnering with patients to improve care is a trend that will be the norm in the next decade.

Working with New Technologies

Technology is a major driver of change in health care. New technology arrives at such an incredible rate that it is impossible to be current in all aspects of the newest and latest advancements. New technology has created more procedures and more effective treatments, and patients want the latest developments. What worked yesterday may or may not be the best option for today. And with each new technology, the workplace environment changes.

New skills are needed to use these technological advances, and retraining is even more of a constant necessity for health-care providers than in previous decades. Health-care providers who enjoy continually learning new procedures will find health-care delivery to be exciting. Others who prefer a more stable work environment may have to opt for some form of career change or position themselves in health-care positions where technology has less of an impact.

Working in Changing Treatment and Recovery Settings

Treatment is moving from hospital-based care to outpatient clinics, extended care facilities, and the home. Procedures that involved several days in the hospital 10 years ago are now often performed as routine outpatient or short-stay care.

> When there is an alternative to long hospital stays, the delivery of care moves outside the hospital.

When there is an alternative to long hospital stays, the delivery of care moves outside the hospital. Increasingly health-care providers are being asked to go into the community instead of making rounds in a clean, comfortable hospital. The workplace for many in health care has changed or will change dramatically.

Adapting to New Ownership and New Structures

The business of health care is changing the ownership of health-care delivery systems. Consolidations, mergers, and acquisitions are in the news every day, and each time one occurs, it brings change to that specific health-care workplace.

Basically these ownership changes are about who pays for health care and how payment occurs. We know that ultimately the consumer pays, but the way in which payment takes place is still being discussed. Will there be an extensive national health-care program that involves the government? Will insurance companies as we know them continue to be involved? Will providers end up owning all the businesses that provide health-care? Will there be new and different kinds of health-care business alliances?

We don't know, and as we have talked with leaders from all facets of the health-care industry, we have not found consensus. What we do know is that these are some of the questions being discussed, and as you know, the answers may well change even further how health care is delivered in this country.

Identifying Change in Health Care

Until these issues get settled, however, we can count on several organizational events continuing:

- Health-care organizations will continue to flatten their structures. There will be fewer managers, and managers will have more to do. People who might have entered health care to move up the ladder will find fewer rungs on that ladder.

- Work will increasingly be accomplished in teams. Already health care is ahead of many other fields in the use of teams, process training, and evaluation. Whether collaborative or self-directed teams emerge is yet to be seen.

- The push will continue to do more with less. Fewer people will be expected to accomplish the same amount of work as before. Efficiencies will be pushed, sometimes beyond the limit. Organizations will experiment with different kinds of work arrangements to see which procedures are the most cost-effective.

Change is a constant for health care, and will be well into the next century.

To sum it all up, change is a constant for health care, and will be well into the next century.

Remember, this is a book about action. It's not enough just to identify the changes taking place in health care. The focus of this book is on making change work for you in the health-care setting.

- You begin by identifying the changes taking place in your organization.

- Next you commit to making that change work for you.

- Then you master the skills that will make you a change expert.

In the following chapter, we'll help you begin to develop those skills by discussing what is already known about change.

Identifying Change in Health Care

Action!

Think about the world in which you work. What are the changes taking place? Are they similar to what's been discussed in Chapter 1. Or are they different? In the spaces below, briefly describe the biggest changes affecting you in each area of work.

	Managing Wellness	Partnering with Patients	New Technologies	Changing Treatment and Recovery	New Ownership and New Settings
Structures					
Individually					
Your Department					
Your Facility					
Your Health-Care Field					

15

Chapter Two

What We Already Know About Change

In Chapter 1, we discussed some of the changes taking place in today's health-care industry. Though dealing with these changes can be challenging, we must remember that the process of change itself is perfectly natural.

> **Each of us has been dealing with change since birth, and by the time we're adults, we've experienced all kinds of changes.**

Each of us has been dealing with change since birth, and by the time we're adults, we've experienced all kinds of changes—learning how to walk, how to talk, how to read; changing from a child to an adolescent to an adult; changing from being taken care of to taking care of ourselves to taking care of others. And of course, change isn't limited to our individual lives. Our environment changes continually as well. Think about the constant change you see in seasons and the weather, cultural trends and fads, customs and protocol.

It's not so surprising then that the health-care workplace has changed considerably in the past few years. In order to develop and implement your own personal strategy for making change work for you in health care, you need to be aware of five basic dynamics about change:

1. Self-chosen change is the easiest.

2. We are what we are because of change.

3. The way work gets done is rapidly changing.

4. Change that affects relationships is the most difficult.

5. Change is constant.

These dynamics have been identified through our research in working with individuals and organizations in change, as well as from the efforts of others like Lyle Schaller. As you read what we already know about change, try to interact with the concepts and words and apply them to your own situation. How have the various change dynamics played out in your work setting? How can you apply a dynamic to your situation now?

What We Already Know About Change

Dynamic 1: Self-Chosen Change Is the Easiest

Change that we choose ourselves is the easiest kind to experience. This is true whether it happens to be organizational change or personal change. When we make the conscious decision to go through some kind of change, we usually understand that it may involve some discomfort. But in making the decision, we also decide to make the best of any stress or unpleasantness the change may bring. We probably weighed the pluses and minuses during our decision-making process and decided to go ahead with the change despite the difficulties.

- When Gina, an R.N. with several years experience in ICCU and a cardiac cath lab, decided to go back to school to become a nurse practitioner, she knew what it would involve. She knew it would mean long hours, considerably less time at home with her husband and two children, and for a few years at least, less time for herself and those who were important to her.

  Gina decided to return to school despite these difficulties. Now part way through, she's learned that the sacrifices were even greater than earlier anticipated. She's tired and hasn't had a full night's sleep in months. Gina has experienced all kinds of changes. "But it was my decision," she says. "In fact, it was our decision. Roger, Sue, and Brad all agreed that I should go for it if that's what I really wanted. Has it been worth it? Yes! Has it taken a lot of sacrifices? Yes! But it's been my choice."

Change that's not of our own choosing, often called *mandated change*, is more difficult to deal with. We often react negatively to change that's imposed on us—sometimes just because someone else made the decision. When a change isn't our decision, we sometimes respond to it with a learned reaction, which is to fight and resist it.

> We often react negatively to change that's imposed on us—sometimes just because someone else made the decision.

We call it a *learned* reaction because the authors believe change is a natural phenomenon. And if change is natural, our first instinct is to make change work. If we resist change, it is because we have been *taught* that people should be stressed when change occurs—we have been *taught* that people should go through a process of anger and denial.

True, there are some changes imposed upon us that are more difficult to deal with than other change. These include the death of a spouse, child, loved one, or patient who has touched us; serious illness; a critical accident; or selling our practice. But the vast majority of change we experience is not negative, and there's absolutely no reason to approach it with anger and denial. After all, we do not talk about anger and denial when a new technology is introduced that increases cures. Organizational change usually is change over which we have little, if

What We Already Know About Change

any, control. We're out of the decision-making loop. Others make the decisions that affect us. But our decision about how to react to organizational change really is our own. After all, we can decide it's unfair, or we can decide it's inconvenient, or we even can decide that the change is positive! What's important to know is that we can learn to make change work for us, even when it's imposed on us and not of our own choice.

■ When Dennis was told his position within a health insurance company was eliminated and he would either have to take a position with less responsibility or exit the company, he wasn't pleased. It was change outside his immediate control.

The only thing Dennis could control was his reaction to the change. And that's what he did. Dennis left the insurance company and within six months secured a new position that fit his skills, drive, and experience in provider relations. "I decided to make the change work for me," he says. "Even though it wasn't my own choosing, I made the commitment to make the change work, and it did!"

Dynamic 2: We Are What We Are Because of Change

When we think about it, the changes we've experienced, self-chosen and imposed upon us, are the things that make us what we are today. We simply are what we are because we've experienced a great deal of change. And that change has had various effects on our lives.

> We simply are what we are because we've experienced a great deal of change. And that change has had various effects on our lives.

■ When Sam's father suddenly died, Sam was angry. "My father died at absolutely the lowest point in my life," Sam says. "I had gone through a divorce and then got fired. I was unemployed, had bills to pay, and kept coming in second in the job interviews. The last time I saw Dad, I was a mess."

Sam's life began to changed for the better, but the disappointment was still there. "Dad never got to see me progress, see things pull back for me, see my first article published or meet the person who is such an important part of my life," he continues. "Relationships mean a lot more to me today than they used to. I learned, and I grew, and I am a better parent and caregiver because of that experience."

Of course, most of the changes that shape us are much less dramatic than Sam's. Kay's experience is similar to many. She tells the story of the day when, as a child, she had "had it with my family." She fixed a peanut butter sandwich, grabbed her little red wagon, and started to run away. But when she got to the corner she had to stop because, "after all, Mom had told me I couldn't cross the street by myself." Shortly Kay's brother showed up, said supper was ready, and they both went home.

What We Already Know About Change

"What fascinated me," Kay reports, "was watching the kids in the next block. I still remember how excited I was the first time I could cross the street by myself. It opened a whole new world that has continued to expand."

Many of us have experienced change that affected the way we provide care to our patients. We all know who makes the worst patient—a caregiver.

- Pam, a nurse, gained a new appreciation for the demands of her patients when she was hospitalized. She developed new and expanded empathy for the frustrations and helplessness of patients. Pam was able to take a new look at the way she cared for her patients, and she was a better caregiver because of her experience.

As these and many other examples point out, we are what we are because of the changes we've already experienced. Those changes aren't always likable or enjoyable. Sometimes they're tragic. But they've shaped us and our actions and reactions, and they've made us what we are.

Dynamic 3: The Way Work Gets Done Is Rapidly Changing

The workplace looks different than it did just a few years ago, not only in health care, but also in all sectors of the economy. The way work gets done is rapidly changing. Many of these changes are the result of technological developments. Others have occurred because of societal changes, global economic changes, and changes in the ways organizations are structured. Here are five ways the workplace is changing:

New Technology

New technology has had a tremendous impact on health care.

As we saw in Chapter 1, new technology has had a tremendous impact on health care. Technology has created new fields, such as nuclear medicine. Procedures that used to be traumatic can now be done through noninvasive procedures. Diagnosis can take place across the Internet using a team of caregivers.

Technology is also drastically changing the way health-care work gets done. In many health-care settings, physicians and nurses have PCs in their examining rooms and enter data immediately rather than relying on dictation or handwritten notes. Caregivers are expected to learn the appropriate software and use their computers for record-keeping functions.

Where will new technology take us? We don't know for sure. What we do know, however, is that the workplace is changing because of it.

What We Already Know About Change

Changing Population

The population of the United States is aging, and the average age of workers will continue to increase. The percentage of workers under age 30 is expected to decline in the next 20 years, and so will the number of workers available for entry-level jobs. The full impact of these changes isn't clear, but they're certain to change the way work gets done.

In health care, we expect to see more patients receiving care from fewer caregivers. Older caregivers, who will still be needed to deliver health care, may or may not accept long hours, weekend work, or an increased patient load. They may look to flex time.

Competition

In the U.S., we've seen a great push for health-care providers to be competitive. As our country struggles with how health-care costs will be paid, the competition between providers will increase.

This competition will focus in two areas:

1. Competition to provide service at reduced costs. Efficiencies will be pushed, sometimes beyond their limits. As we've already seen, pushing some efficiencies, such as length of stay after childbirth, are not always popular or medically sound.

2. As costs are reduced, we project a renewed interest in patient satisfaction and customer service. The challenge is to provide the kind of care that has high patient loyalty.

Outside of health care, companies struggle to remain competitive with their foreign counterparts. The need to be competitive has resulted in mergers, acquisitions, consolidations, and of course, layoffs. The push seems to be for the highest quality service at the absolute lowest cost, regardless of source. As large investors demand higher returns on their investments, they are increasingly less concerned about where their returns come from.

Corporate purchasing personnel know this and continually look for ways to cut costs. If a foreign supplier can produce a similar or better product at a lower cost, it likely will be favored with the purchasing contract. The bottom line: Cost of goods matters more than their place of origin. Cost cutting will continue to be a hot topic and will definitely continue to affect the way work gets done.

> In the U.S., we've seen a great push for health-care providers to be competitive.

What We Already Know About Change

Organizational Structure

> Businesses, nonprofit groups, and government agencies have been flattening their organizational structures for some time.

Businesses, nonprofit groups, and government agencies have been flattening their organizational structures for some time. The same holds true in health care. One midwestern hospital that once had 9 vice presidents, 16 directors, and 35 managers now has 2 vice presidents and 8 directors, 20 managers, and 20 team leaders.

In most organizations there are now fewer midlevel managers, which means there is less opportunity for advancement: More and more people will have to accept lateral moves instead of making a continual climb up the corporate ladder. Some people even are saying that the goal of climbing the corporate ladder has become unrealistic and out of date. A new paradigm about careers and work will instead begin to emerge.

Career Moves

The days of having just one job with one company ended some time ago. Instead, people begin their careers in one field and may move to several other fields and areas of expertise before retirement.

"In health care, staff members need to be aware of what they do best and what they most enjoy doing," states Judy Seiler, R.N., manager of training and development at Scottsdale Healthcare, Scottsdale, AZ. "As health care reorganizes and adds new technology, jobs will vanish, and people will need to take another kind of position to remain working within health care." Knowing one's own skills, Seiler asserts, will become essential if a person wishes to stay employed in health care.

Instead of having just one career, a worker may contract with a company to perform a set of tasks. Once those tasks—and the worker's assignment—are completed, the worker negotiates another contract with perhaps a different company for a new set of tasks. What will the eventual impact be? We can't know for sure, but what we do know is that the way work gets done is changing!

What We Already Know About Change

Dynamic 4: Change That Affects Relationships Is the Most Difficult

Although technological or organizational change often takes place rapidly, change that involves interpersonal relationships tends to take longer. A department can be reorganized—even downsized—in a very short time. A year later, however, the people in that department still may talk about the changes they went through and the impact of those changes.

> **Even when it may seem all right to change how we do our work, we still may resist changes that affect the people with whom we work.**

Even when it may seem all right to change how we do our work, we still may resist changes that affect the people with whom we work. The more people like working together, the more difficult it is for them to go through a personnel change. This may explain, in part, why productivity typically increases when a company makes an announcement that it's closing a facility or eliminating a work group or closing a department. If the employees have an especially good working relationship, they tend to increase their productivity.

As one person explains, "We worked harder, hoping that if the decision makers saw how productive we were, they wouldn't go through with the changes. Then we all could continue working together."

The dynamic seems to go like this: If you don't enjoy the people with whom you work, you're ready for any kind of change that will put you in contact with coworkers you may like better. You welcome change, applaud it, anticipate it. But if you already like the people with whom you work, it's not as easy to go through organizational change. It takes longer to adjust, to regain confidence in the organization, and to trust your new coworkers.

If you perform your job primarily by yourself, having to change the way you work may be little more than an inconvenience. You may have to learn new procedures or tasks, but the overall impact of the change is minimal. But if your work depends on others, as it does so extensively in health care, and the quality of those working relationships is high, any organizational change will have a much greater impact.

It will take more time and energy for you to adjust. After all, you'll have to develop new relationships, and you probably wonder how long it will take to trust these new people. When an employee leaves a group of coworkers who enjoyed working with him or her, the remaining employees experience a sense of personal loss. A kind of grieving process sets in, and it takes longer for them to adjust to the change than if the work unit had been left intact.

What We Already Know About Change

Dynamic 5: Change Is Constant

Whether we like it or not, the pace of organizational change will increase rather than decrease. There will be more changes in the next 10 years than in the past 10. Change will be more frequent, more comprehensive, more compressed.

This should be no surprise to us, though. We've seen that change is a natural phenomenon that is constantly taking place in and around us. And since change is a natural phenomenon, you have the natural ability to make change work. In the following chapters, you will have the opportunity to increase your skills in making change work in health care.

Action!

Take some time to reflect on what you've read in Chapter 2. What parts of this chapter had the most impact on you? Why? How? Take some time to reflect, and write a note to yourself describing the insights from this chapter that have the most meaning for you.

_____

_____

_____

_____

Chapter Three

Why Everyone Doesn't React to Change the Same Way

You've probably noticed that many of your coworkers react differently to organizational change than you do.

As your health-care organization has experienced change, you've probably noticed that many of your coworkers react differently to organizational change than you do. If you kept track of your observations, you may have noticed that during an organizational change some of your coworkers wanted to know more about the change and why it was necessary, others wanted to know the details of how things were going to be reorganized, and still others seemed energized by the prospect of the change.

As you listened to individuals react to organizational change, you probably kept hearing words and phrases such as:

- "Why?"
- "Yeah, but . . ."
- "Why not?"
- "Well, show me!"

You probably also noticed that some seemed to ask "Why?" one day and "Why not?" the next.

The system that answers the most questions and provides the most sensible information about how individuals react to change is based on the concept of *conation*. This chapter will introduce you to conation, explain why people react to change in different ways, and describe the four major ways people naturally react to change, using the information identified and developed by Kathy Kolbe.

Kolbe's concept of conation provides a reasonable, practical, and highly useful approach to actions and the natural ways people get things done. It will help you understand the various actions and reactions of your coworkers as they go through organizational change. After all, actions speak louder than words.

Why Everyone Doesn't React to Change the Same Way

Conation: How We Naturally Get Things Done

Ancient philosophers talked about three parts of the mind: the parts that govern thinking, feeling, and doing. The thinking part is referred to as intelligence, or the *cognitive* part of the mind. The feeling part is referred to as personality, or the *affective* part of the mind. And the doing part is referred to as instinct, or the *conative* part of the mind.

> The "doing" part of the mind is referred to as instinct, or the *conative* part of the mind.

The conative part of the mind has to do with:

- How we naturally and instinctively get things done.
- Actions, not feelings.
- The natural instincts each person has for striving to accomplish things.

The concept of conation was rediscovered in our country by management specialist Kathy Kolbe. After spending several years researching the subject, Kolbe developed a system to help people understand their natural conative talents.

The Kolbe Conative Action Modes™

Kolbe's research indicated that there are four separate action modes out of which people naturally and instinctively get things done—like reacting to organizational change in health care. Kolbe calls these four action modes *Fact Finder, Follow Thru, Quick Start,* and *Implementor.* Her research also indicated that each person has natural talents in all four action modes, but usually more energy in one or two modes and less in the others.

Kolbe also asserts that no action mode is better than any other. It's not better to be a Fact Finder or a Quick Start than it is to be a Follow Thru or an Implementor. Each action mode makes contributions to every organization, and all action modes are needed for total effectiveness.

Kolbe's research found that our individual conative talent isn't a matter of heredity or environment. Instead, it's like a thumbprint—it just is! And it doesn't change over time. A person's conative makeup is basically the same at age 55 as it was at age 5. It may be more understood and appreciated at 55, but it was there all along. Kolbe's research also found that there are no conative instincts that are just for men or just for women.

When we use our natural talents and have the freedom to do things the way we instinctively do them, we're energized and fully productive, and we enjoy what we're doing. When we have to work "against the grain"—not the way we'd naturally do things—we become stressed.

Why Everyone Doesn't React to Change the Same Way

To help you understand the various ways people respond to change, here are descriptions of the four action modes identified by Kolbe. Although only the Kolbe A Index (see page 35 for more information) can specifically identify your conative makeup, you can gain an appreciation of your conative instincts by reviewing these descriptions. As you read the description for each action mode:

- Think about yourself and how you naturally get things done.
- Think about others with whom you work and how you've observed them get things done.

You'll find it helpful to circle or highlight those words that seem to describe your most natural actions.

Fact Finder

Fact Finder is the action mode out of which a person naturally and instinctively probes and gathers information.

This is the action mode out of which a person naturally and instinctively probes and gathers information. It is out of this action mode that a person is:

- Practical
- Realistic
- Specific
- Detailed
- Objective
- Thorough
- Tactful
- Deliberate
- Investigative
- Inquisitive
- Informed
- Appropriate

A person with a good deal of natural energy in the Fact Finder action mode learns from history, appreciates what did and did not work before, and instinctively gathers information. This person doesn't like to be pushed to do anything until enough information is at hand in order to do the task well. Appropriateness and thoroughness are key factors for a person with natural energy in the Fact Finder mode.

When a Fact Finder is given a task, this person will first stop and gather all the information deemed necessary to get the job done. Fact Finders are at their best when they can weigh the pros and cons and have time to make a well-thought-out decision.

Why Everyone Doesn't React to Change the Same Way

The basic perspective of the Fact Finder is on the past, and a person with high intensity in this action mode thinks in terms of tradition and what is and is not appropriate. This person remembers what did and did not work before in similar situations and views a new task from the perspective of what worked before in similar, though not always identical, situations. Background information and thoroughness are important to the Fact Finder.

People who have a good deal of natural energy in the Fact Finder mode typically respond to change by analyzing it and asking "Why?"

People who have a good deal of natural energy in the Fact Finder mode typically respond to change by analyzing it and asking "Why?" It isn't that they're against change or that they fight it—they just need to know why the change is necessary, what the change involves, how it relates to what did and didn't work before, and what to expect. Then they need time to think about it. If the change is considered by the Fact Finder to be "appropriate," the Fact Finder typically will be a strong supporter of it.

Without enough information, Fact Finders will become stressed during organizational change. If the company doesn't provide enough information about the change, the Fact Finder either will try to find the answers or listen to rumors.

Fact Finders make an important contribution to organizational change by continuing to ask the question "Why?" and pushing decision makers to provide enough information to let employees know what will be happening, why the change is important, and what future expectations will be.

Action!

Review the words and phrases you have underlined or highlighted. Do you think you have a lot of instinctive energy in the Fact Finder action mode? a moderate amount? a lesser amount? Are you a person who naturally researches and gathers information? who wants things to be appropriate? who frequently asks, "Why?"

Remember, each action mode makes important contributions. It's not better to be a Fact Finder than a Follow Thru or a Quick Start than an Implementor. It's just the way people are.

Why Everyone Doesn't React to Change the Same Way

Follow Thru

> *Follow Thru* is the action mode out of which a person naturally and instinctively coordinates and organizes.

This is the action mode out of which a person naturally and instinctively coordinates and organizes. It is out of this mode that a person is:

- Efficient
- Systematic
- Consistent
- Methodical
- Coordinated
- Disciplined
- Dependable
- Theoretical
- Structured
- Concise
- Meticulous
- Organized

A person with a good deal of natural energy in the Follow Thru action mode thinks in terms of patterns and is able to organize almost anything: time, people, desktops, clothes, work, schedules, paper, numbers, budgets, or events. Efficiency and consistency are key factors for a person with high intensity in the Follow Thru action mode.

When a Follow Thru is given a task and is free to complete it his or her own way, this person will think in terms of organization and order. This person wants to fit everything together, coordinate it, and place it in proper perspective. When Follow Thrus organize time or work, they do it in terms of what needs to be done first, second, third, and so on. Follow Thrus also want to stay with their original schedule and sequence. Interruptions, unless scheduled or anticipated, usually are stressful. Follow Thrus are at their best when they can make a decision in a nonrushed, organized manner.

> Follow Thru wants to know how the change will fit into the overall scheme of things and particularly how it will fit into the system that's already in place.

The basic perspective of a Follow Thru is integration of past, present, and future. Follow Thrus strive to view things within the context of the whole situation. The person with a high intensity in the Follow Thru mode may outwardly appear to resist change. The person will make comments such as, "Yeah, this may be necessary, but . . ." The yeah-buts often are misinterpreted. It's not that the person actually resists change—just that the Follow Thru wants to know how the change will fit into the overall scheme of things and particularly how it will fit into the system that's already in place. The Follow Thru needs time to think about the change.

Without an agenda of how the change is to take place (what will happen first, next, and so on) and how the change will affect daily routines, the Follow Thru will be stressed during an organizational change. Structure and security are important to Follow Thrus, and if

Why Everyone Doesn't React to Change the Same Way

the structure is changed without adequate preparation, threatening job security, this person will be stressed.

Because the Follow Thru likes to have his or her day structured—and structured in a consistent way—organizational change can stress the Follow Thru until new patterns are in place. Asking Follow Thrus to do something one way today and a different way tomorrow will be stressful.

Follow Thrus make an important contribution to organizational change by striving to keep balance. Because of their natural instinct to organize, they will strive to bring order out of chaos and find ways to make certain that the things that need doing actually get done.

Action!
Review the words you've underlined or highlighted. Do you think you have a lot of instinctive energy in the Follow Thru action mode? a moderate amount? a lesser amount? Are you a person who naturally likes to organize people, papers, numbers, or work? who makes a list of what needs to get done and then follows that list? who frequently says, "'Yeah, but . . . ?"

Quick Start

Quick Start is the action mode out of which a person naturally and instinctively innovates, takes risks, is spontaneous, and quickly moves from project to project.

This is the action mode out of which a person naturally and instinctively innovates, takes risks, is spontaneous, and quickly moves from project to project. It is out of this action mode that a person is:

- Inventive
- Intuitive
- Flexible
- Fluent
- Imaginative
- Adventurous
- Decisive
- Spontaneous
- Conceptual
- A deal maker
- A risk taker
- A promoter

A person with a good deal of natural energy in the Quick Start action mode has many things going on at the same time and may be viewed by others as bouncing off the walls. This person naturally looks for new ways to do things and often is persuasive in promoting an idea, agenda, service, or product.

● Why Everyone Doesn't React to Change the Same Way

When given a task, the Quick Start naturally begins thinking in terms of innovations and new ways to do what's been done before. Quick Starts work best out of a sense of challenge and, because they typically handle several things at once, appreciate the pressure of deadlines.

The basic perspective of the Quick Start is that of the future. Quick Starts naturally think in terms of what's ahead and of possibilities. Being instinctively conceptual, they can envision the big picture without getting bogged down with details. They usually think ahead of themselves and others. The freedom to change things is important to the Quick Start.

> **People who have a good deal of natural energy in the Quick Start action mode respond to change by promoting it.**

People who have a good deal of natural energy in the Quick Start action mode respond to change by promoting it. They are the change agents. Quick Starts will be advocates of change and encourage others to "try it, you'll like it!" Natural risk takers, Quick Starts are ready to try just about anything that makes sense at the moment and will evaluate it after they see how it all works out.

Quick Starts especially can become stressed during organizational change. They will have a difficult time when they aren't involved in coming up with the new alternatives or when the proposed change doesn't take place quickly enough for them. Quick Starts also will become stressed if the change imposes a structured way of doing things on them.

Quick Starts make an important contribution to organizational change not only by coming up with new ways to approach old tasks, but also by encouraging others to see the benefits of the change. Quick Starts will be the ones who say, "Hey, why not?" or "Let's give it a try," or "What have we got to lose?" Quick Starts thrive in the midst of change. They live for change.

Action!

Review the words you've underlined or highlighted. Do you think you have a lot of instinctive energy in the Quick Start action mode? a moderate amount? a lesser amount? Are you a person who is naturally intuitive, flexible, and willing to try different things? who frequently asks, "Why not?" who works best under pressure?

Why Everyone Doesn't React to Change the Same Way ●

Implementor

This is the action mode out of which a person naturally and instinctively works with his or her hands. It is out of this action mode that a person is:

> *Implementor* is the action mode out of which a person naturally and instinctively works with his or her hands.

- Mechanical
- Tangible
- A builder
- Tactile
- Hands-on
- A crafter
- Technical
- A demonstrator
- A fabricator

People with a good deal of natural energy in the Implementor action mode do things with their hands or work with tools and machines. They are typically concerned about the quality of what is produced. These people learn by doing and are naturally able to visualize space and how best to make use of it. Remember, Implementors work with their hands. This action mode has nothing to do with implementing an idea or assignment.

When given a task, an Implementor will stop and visualize what needs to happen. The Implementors will then gather all the proper tools and materials needed to complete the task and then will set about completing it. Implementors are at their best when they have time to construct solutions and produce tangible and visual results that meet their standards of quality.

The basic perspective of the Implementor is on the present; he or she thinks in terms of the here and now. Implementors want to make sure that whatever they build will endure, so that the quality of today will be available in the future. They see no need to describe in words what they can present in a model. People with high intensity in the Implementor action mode use props to help them express their ideas to others.

People with a high level of natural energy in the Implementor action mode often aren't as verbal as people with natural energy in the other modes. Since language is conceptual and abstract, to do well with language one also must do well with conceptual and abstract activities. But because Implementors work from the perspective of the present, the specific, and the here and now, they don't approach activities from the perspective of the abstract. It's not that they can't verbally communicate, but that they tend to communicate in specifics. For an Implementor, actions truly do speak louder than words.

● Why Everyone Doesn't React to Change the Same Way

> **People who have a good deal of natural energy in the Implementor action mode typically respond to change with a concern for continued quality and continuity.**

People who have a good deal of natural energy in the Implementor action mode typically respond to change with a concern for continued quality and continuity. Their concerns tend to focus on the continued opportunity to produce a quality product with the right equipment. If the change involves downgrading the materials or tools used to produce the product, they will resist it. If, on the other hand, the change involves upgrading materials or tools, they will support the change.

Because people with high intensity in the Implementor action mode tend to be nonverbal, the stress they may experience from change isn't always easy to notice. Implementors tend to keep things to themselves; they use few words to communicate their concerns. It's easier for Implementors to talk about personal reactions or feelings when they're working at something with their hands or when they're walking or hiking.

Implementors make an important contribution to organizational change by focusing on the importance of having the right space, the right materials, and the right equipment to produce or provide a quality product.

Action!
Review the words you've underlined or highlighted. Do you think you have a lot of instinctive energy in the Implementor action mode? a moderate amount? a lesser amount? Are you a person who naturally works with his or her hands or with machines or tools? who is sometimes nonverbal? who says, "Show me, don't tell me"?

Combinations

As you've read this information, you may have thought, "I'm not exactly like any one action mode. I seem to be more like a little bit of each, but with more intensity in two of them." You may be right. People have instinctive energy in all four action modes, but usually have higher intensities in one or sometimes two of them. When people have higher levels of natural energy in two action modes, combinations occur.

- ■ A person may have high intensity in the Quick Start mode as well as the Fact Finder mode. When experiencing organizational change, this person instinctively will promote it and think of even more new ways to get things done. Then the person will stop and ask for more information. If the levels of intensity are fairly equal, the person will go back and forth between supporting the change and wanting to know more about it. It may seem to others that the person sometimes says "Why not?" in the morning and "Why?" in the afternoon.

Why Everyone Doesn't React to Change the Same Way

■ A person with a good deal of natural energy in the Follow Thru and Implementor action modes will respond to organizational change first by wanting to know how it all fits together and then how the change will fit into the existing structure. The person will want some kind of visualization, like a three-dimensional model or a graph or chart. It may seem as if the person says "Yeah, but . . ." one moment and "Show me" the next.

Remember, people have talents in each of the four conative action modes. Most, however, have much stronger levels of energy in one, and sometimes two, of the modes. It's how we are. Some of us naturally gather information, while others naturally organize, innovate, or work with their hands.

Conative Strengths and Organizational Change

> People react to organizational change according to their natural instincts.

People react to organizational change according to their natural instincts, their conative style. That's why some people respond to organizational change one way and others respond another way. Now that you've been introduced to the third part of the mind—the conative part—and have seen how people instinctively and naturally get things done, you know that everyone doesn't react to organizational change in the same way:

- **The Fact Finder** instinctively wants enough information about the organizational change to be certain it will be successful, is appropriate to the situation, and is consistent with what's worked before.

- **The Follow Thru** instinctively wants the organizational change to be well organized and introduced in a way that helps everyone understand and accept it, and will help ensure that everything fits together.

- **The Quick Start** will help promote the change and will encourage others to "try it, you'll like it!"

- **The Implementor** wants to maintain quality and ensure that the right tools or equipment and adequate space are available to get the job done well.

Why Everyone Doesn't React to Change the Same Way

> **Action!**
> Now that you've read through the descriptions of each action mode, you may have a sense of where your natural talents and instincts are. If so, take a sheet of paper and write a brief description. If you aren't able to describe you natural talents and instincts after this brief introduction, you may want to read one of Kolbe's books. See page 35 for more information.

Kathy Kolbe defines success as "the freedom to be yourself." When a person is free to be himself or herself, to do things naturally and instinctively, that person is productive, creative, and satisfied. In other words, successful. Work isn't difficult, but enjoyable because the person is able to do it in the way that's most natural.

But there's a tradeoff. If you want to be successful, free to be yourself and respond to organizational change naturally and instinctively, then you must do one more thing. You must acknowledge that others will have different instincts than you do and will naturally respond to organizational change in different ways than you do. We know that in any organization, all people are not just Fact Finders or Quick Starts. There's a variety.

As you can see, all conative action modes are helpful when it comes to designing and responding to organizational change. When you understand your own natural and instinctive talents, appreciate the natural strengths you bring to any situation, and respect the natural instincts of others, you set in motion the energy to make change work for you!

Why Everyone Doesn't React to Change the Same Way

Action!

Now that you've read through the descriptions of the four action modes, you may have a sense of where your natural talents and instincts are, as well as the natural talents of those with whom you work. If so, write a brief description of yourself and key coworkers in the space below.

_____

_____

_____

_____

If you aren't able to describe your natural talents and instincts, you may want to read one of Kolbe's books, listed below.

For more information about conation and the Kolbe Concept™, read either of Kathy Kolbe's books: *The Conative Connection: Uncovering the Link Between Who You Are and How You Perform* (Addison Wesley, 1990) and *Pure Instinct: Business' Untapped Resource* (Times Books/Random House, 1993).

Kolbe Concept™ and Kolbe Conative Action Modes™ are registered trademarks of KolbeCorp Inc., Phoenix, Arizona. Copyrighted material used by permission.

Chapter Four

Guiding Your Team's Reaction to Change

Now that we've seen why everyone doesn't react to change the same way, let's shift our attention from the individual to the work unit. The work unit can be a work team of several people, a work unit such as a cardiac rehab unit, or even an entire department, such as med-surg or admitting.

As we've seen, when individuals are free to be themselves, they react to change based on their conative strengths. Work units, however, tend to have other characteristics in responding to organizational change. We have found that with no interventions, work units react to change in a fairly predictable pattern. When you know and understand how work teams follow this pattern, these reactions won't blindside you or catch you by surprise.

> **With no interventions, work units react to change in a fairly predictable pattern.**

You will also be able to stop and ask yourself, "How does this work team really want to react to the pending change or the change we just went through?" As a work team answers this question, the team takes control of their collective reactions and makes change work.

As illustrated in Figure 1, teams of any size or description typically go through five stages when dealing with change:

1. Positioning
2. Uncertainty
3. Clarification
4. Focus
5. Acceptance

These changes are normal, so there's nothing wrong with your work team if it exhibits these reactions.

We've learned that typically, each work unit will go through each stage. Work units may vary in how long they remain in one stage or another, however, depending on the makeup of the unit and on how well the change is being managed. And throughout all of this, there is the ever-present reality of rumors.

Guiding Your Team's Reaction to Change

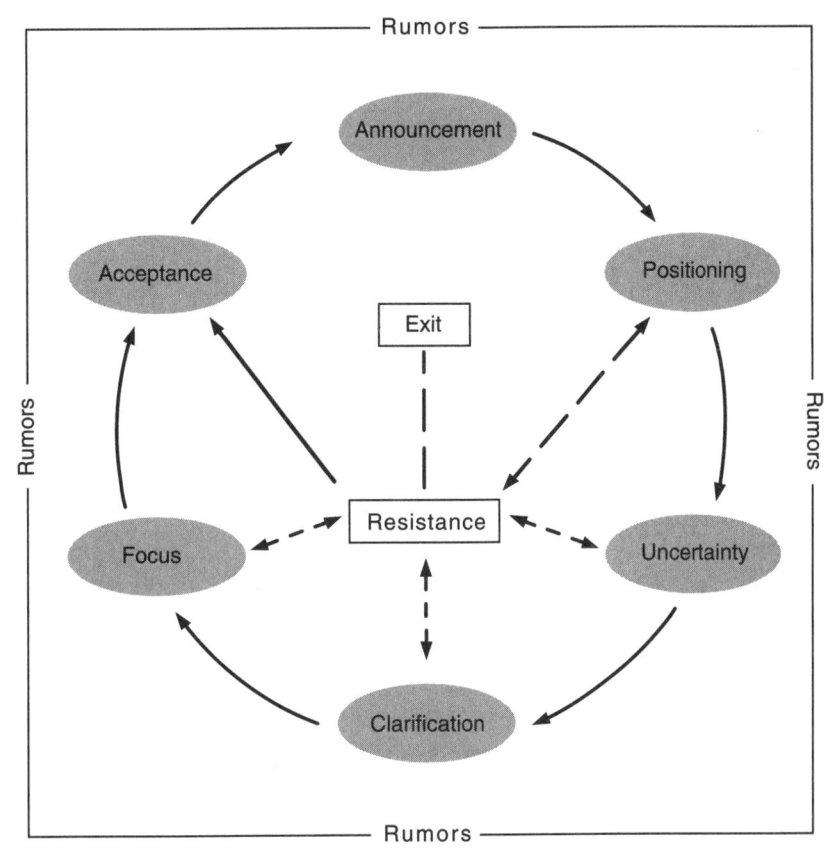

Figure 1—Organization Change Reaction Cycle

Setting the Stage: Rumors and the Announcement

Rumors exist even before a formal announcement is made about any reorganization or change. Some will be fairly accurate; others will be totally wrong. Some people will listen to the rumors, particularly the gloom-and-doom predictions; others will pay them little attention.

Because of rumors, the organization's formal *announcement* usually isn't a total surprise. The specifics of the announcement may be a surprise, but in general, earlier discussions among employees will have anticipated much of what the announcement will say. The announcement is quickly followed by the first stage.

> **Because of rumors, the organization's formal *announcement* usually isn't a total surprise.**

Stage 1: Positioning

The formal announcement is quickly followed by a time of *positioning*. Work units step back and take an initial position on the announced change. There may be some jockeying as various work teams attempt to position themselves for what each perceives to be the best response. These positions will vary from unit to unit and are determined by the key influencers within each team.

Guiding Your Team's Reaction to Change

When the organizational change involves only a single team, there is still jockeying among the team members to see who will influence the total group. Whoever wins will set the stage for how others in the group will respond to the change. Though individuals will vary in their particular positions, each work team typically comes to its own collective stand about the organizational change. These positions usually fall into the following categories:

> Though individuals will vary in their particular positions, each work team typically comes to its own collective stand about the organizational change.

- ◆ **Relief**
  For some work teams, there is a sigh of relief—as if collectively the group says, "Finally, at least we know what's going to happen." Many people don't like living with a question mark, and rumors can be unsettling. For these work units, dealing with the known—even if they don't like it—is easier than dealing with the unknown.

- ◆ **Anger**
  For some work teams, the position toward the announcement is one of anger. It's as if the group collectively says, "How dare you do this to us! We're upset, angry, and mad, and somehow we'll get even." The anger can manifest itself in lack of cooperation, decline in productivity, general doom-and-gloom behavior by the unit as a whole, and even sabotage.

- ◆ **Anxiety**
  Some work teams respond to the announcement with anxiety. "What great tragedy will happen next?" they seem to ask. It's as if they're looking back over their shoulders all the time, waiting for something else to happen. Because of their anxiety, they're unable to see anything positive in the announcement.

- ◆ **Wait and see**
  Some work teams position themselves with the cautious "Let's wait and see how this works out" response. They typically don't try to block whatever change is taking place, nor do they fight it. But they aren't necessarily enthusiastic supporters, either. A work unit that positions itself with a wait-and-see attitude still can be influenced by others—other work units or company supervisors and managers. The successful influencer is the one with the most appealing message.

- ◆ **Opportunity**
  Many work teams position themselves to see primarily the opportunities that come with organizational change. They support the change and tend to talk among themselves and with other teams about its potential benefits. A work unit that supports the change can help other units modify their initial positions, particularly if it's well liked and respected and perceived as influential with the new decision makers.

Guiding Your Team's Reaction to Change

Regardless of its size, a work team's first reaction to an announcement of organizational change is to position itself in terms of its response. And the way the change is announced—and the way influencers react to the announcement—can sway work teams either way.

Stage 2: Uncertainty

Positioning is quickly followed by *uncertainty*. In many instances, uncertainty about what the announcement really means sets in before the end of the day. People ask questions like:

- Will it have an impact on me?
- Will I still have a job?
- Will my friends still have jobs?
- Will I have new coworkers? a new boss?
- Will I have to move to a new location?
- Who's making decisions?
- What do these decision makers know about me?
- Who has power?
- Who no longer has power?
- Will I have to take a cut in pay?

Uncertainty is fueled by not having answers to questions like these.

> **People need to understand that in any organizational change, it's impossible for the announcement to include all of the specific details and address all the implications of what the change really means.**

People need to understand that in any organizational change, it's impossible for the announcement to include all of the specific details and address all the implications of what the change really means. Sometimes even the key decision makers don't know what all of the implications will be. It just takes time to work everything out, and during that time, there will be uncertainty.

People often grow up with the notion that all executives, administrators, and top-level managers know everything. They are all-wise. They are natural leaders. And they don't make mistakes. Not so!

In any organizational change, including change in health-care organizations, management contributes to the uncertainty. Management is trying to deal with all aspects of the change. Like employees, decision makers experience uncertainty and confusion. They may seem to say one thing one day and come back the next and say something completely different. Nothing seems consistent.

Guiding Your Team's Reaction to Change

For some employees, this time of uncertainty is just too much. They either decide they don't have to put up with it, or they decide that it's more than they can tolerate. They begin to resist, and might ultimately exit. For people who don't necessarily like change, this time of uncertainty can be very difficult.

Stage 3: Clarification

Uncertainty finally gives way to a sense of *clarification*. Some of the issues that are clarified at this stage include:

- Expectations
- Leadership roles
- Procedures
- Benefits
- Promotions
- Employee downsizing
- Pay procedures

> **Employees now begin to understand their new roles in the changing organization, who has power and who doesn't, and what decision makers think of their work teams.**

Management becomes more consistent. Employees now begin to understand their new roles in the changing organization, who has power and who doesn't, and what decision makers think of their work teams.

Organizational structure becomes clearer, and management's expectations of employees are also clarified. If a new organizational culture is promoted, employees begin to understand what that new culture is all about. Each work team that goes through organizational change will also have its own areas for which it seeks clarification.

How long does it take to go from uncertainty to clarification? It depends. If top management understands change and how to manage it, it may not take long.

Guiding Your Team's Reaction to Change

Stage 4: Focus

Clarification is followed by a time of *focus*. The questions and issues raised during the periods of confusion and clarification have been resolved. If there have been changes in leadership, the new leaders are in place and in charge.

At this stage, management's visions of the health-care organization and its direction are clear. These visions may be the same as they were before, or different. But there is no uncertainty as to what they are, and management shares these visions—the focus—with employees. The expectations for employees are also clear. People know their roles, what is and is not expected of them, and how they are to get things done. Meeting these new expectations may involve a considerable amount of change—or not much at all.

Employees may or may not like the new focus. But at least the direction has been set: There's no more living with a question mark.

Stage 5: Acceptance

Acceptance is the final stage of the change process. During this stage, employees may react in one of three ways:

- **Acceptance with enthusiasm**
  Employees who accept all aspects of the organizational change with enthusiasm now are energized by what has taken place. They like the new direction, the new procedures, and the new leaders. They buy into the new challenges, and their work reflects their new enthusiasm.

- **Acceptance with caution**
  Employees who accept the organizational change with caution still have a wait-and-see attitude. They may like some aspects of the change, but hesitate to endorse all of it. They may like some of the new direction, but can't bring themselves to enthusiastically support it. They decide to wait and see what happens. In the meantime, they get their work done, usually within the range of expectation but seldom better than that. Because people don't like to live with a question mark, these employees will either move on to acceptance with enthusiasm or acceptance with indifference.

- **Acceptance with indifference**
  Employees who accept change with indifference do so because "it's only a job." Their enthusiasm for their work may wane, their willingness to do extra work may be nonexistent, and they may just barely accomplish enough to keep from being fired. They may not intentionally sabotage what the work unit and the health-care

Guiding Your Team's Reaction to Change

organization are trying to accomplish, but they certainly don't add anything to the workplace environment. They are neither fun to be with nor fun to work with. Some will stay in this stage until they retire; they're the people about whom others say, "He retired several months ago, but he just hasn't left yet." The rest either move on to another job, exit, get fired for poor performance, or sometimes move to acceptance with caution and maybe even acceptance with enthusiasm.

There is yet another way in which work teams can react to organizational change: resistance and exit.

Resistance and Exit

Just as rumors surround the reaction patterns of work units that go through change, there also is the dynamic of *resistance and exit*. You'll notice that there are broken lines leading to the resistance box in the center of the Organization Change Reaction Cycle illustration on page 37. At every stage, individual employees, and sometimes entire work teams, can move into resistance.

> **At every stage, individual employees, and sometimes entire work teams, can move into resistance.**

Resistance can take many different forms, including:

◆ Reacting negatively to all that is said and done.

◆ Refusing to go along with new policies and/or procedures.

◆ Becoming difficult to work with.

◆ Becoming sullen or silent.

◆ Attempting to convince others to resist the changes.

One of two things will happen to those in resistance: Either they will exit on their own, or they'll return to the usual reaction pattern. Ultimately, unless they exit, they'll move on to some form of acceptance.

Guiding Your Team's Reaction to Change

Guiding Your Team's Reaction

We have just described the ways that work teams *typically* react to organizational change, but keep in mind *it doesn't always have to be that way!* What we've learned over the years is that when work teams get together and decide how they want to react to change, they do not have to follow the cycle.

> **When work teams get together and decide how they want to react to change, they do not have to follow the cycle.**

■ Sharon was head of nursing services for a medium-size hospital that became part of a statewide health system. The new system instituted a push for all kinds of efficiencies and a major reorganization. Sharon led her management team in a lengthy discussion of the Change Reaction Cycle. Then she asked one more question: "If we could react to the reorganization any way we wanted to, how would we react?"

The group really struggled with their answer, Sharon reports. "Finally, they agreed that what they really wanted to do was make the change work. They didn't want to resist it, but they wanted more information, so they asked for it. Once they had the information about what the new organization was to accomplish, they could do what they wanted to do—support it!"

Because of the personal values that led many health-care professionals into their field, team members may not easily jump from Announcement to Acceptance during organizational change. They may want to consider many variables, such as quality of patient care. But we've learned that when a work team decides to use their conative strengths to react to change, and to move to Acceptance as quickly as possible, it happens.

Action!

How has your work unit previously reacted to change? Is it similar to or different from other work units in your organization? Did it help or hinder the change? Write a brief summary in the space below.

_____

_____

_____

_____

Guiding Your Team's Reaction to Change

Action! *(continued)*

Now ask yourself, "How would I *prefer* my work unit react to change?" Write your description below.

_____

_____

_____

_____

What are the skills you will need in order to guide your team to react to change the way you want it to react? List those skills below. Here's a hint: The next several chapters include many strategies that can help you make change work for you.

_____

_____

_____

_____

Chapter Five

Managing Stress Effectively

Even if you don't want it to, change within your health-care organization can result in stress. There are many reasons why we experience stress during organizational change. They include:

- Hesitating about changing old habits.

- Having to leave your friends from the work unit.

- Undergoing a great deal of change in a short period of time.

- Learning new procedures.

- Having too much to do with too little time and too few resources to do it.

> **Whatever the cause of your stress, there are ways to manage it.**

Whatever the cause of your stress, there are ways to manage it. In fact, by the time you're an adult, you've learned all kinds of ways to manage stress. You've also learned that some strategies work better than others. What's important is to identify the strategies that work for you so you can *effectively* manage any stress that occurs because of organizational change.

The strategies that follow come from people who've been where you are now—in the midst of an organizational change. They have been used successfully by people in health care, from pharmacists to R.N.s to M.D.s to dietary assistants.

As you read about these strategies and practice them on your own, remember that managing the stress that is a result of organizational change is part of making change work. Not every strategy is useful for everybody, but we guarantee that you'll find several strategies in the next pages that will increase your stress-management skills. You'll discover that these strategies help you feel better—more energized, more confident, and more able to deal successfully with each day's events!

Managing Stress Effectively

Strategy 1: Use Your Endorphins

You're aware of endorphins, those chemicals released by the body that have positive effects on mood, outlook, and ability to deal with stress. These are the natural chemicals that our bodies release after a period of several different kinds of activities. These chemicals reduce stress, relieve pain, and in general simply make us feel better!

> *Endorphins reduce stress, relieve pain, and in general simply make us feel better!*

Researchers have studied endorphin production in joggers and runners. After running for a while, these people begin to experience a "runner's high" caused by the release of endorphins. Result? They feel better.

Running isn't the only activity that encourages endorphin production. There are many other ways, including other types of exercise, music, and laughter.

Exercise

The single most effective way to reduce stress is through exercise. This is the one strategy that is almost universally effective—everyone benefits from it. And you don't have to be a natural athlete or spend a lot of money to take advantage of it. Sure, you can join a fitness center with all kinds of exercise machines or invest in home exercise equipment. But those aren't the only options, as others have reported:

- "When I get stressed, I go for a walk. After 30 minutes, I begin to feel better."

- "I have some weights at home that I use. After I learned how to use them, I found that a 30-minute workout three times a week does wonders to keep me smiling."

- "My yard is my exercise. In fact, I've realized that I planned my yard so that I have to work in it at least an hour each evening during the growing seasons. It keeps me stable."

- "Exercise videos help because they give me some direction, and my neighbor helped me understand how important it is to stretch out and get ready."

It's not how you exercise but the fact that you do it that's important! Exercise for 20 to 30 minutes, and you'll naturally feel better.

● Managing Stress Effectively

Music

Music can be like exercise for many people. After listening to whatever kind of music makes them feel good, their bodies begin to produce endorphins, and they naturally feel better. Their stress levels are reduced, their moods improve, and change becomes manageable. The nice thing about music is that you can listen to it on the way to work, during your working day, on the way home, and during your off-hours time.

What kinds of music are best for relieving stress? There's no easy answer. We've found that some people like rock, others find that easy-listening music relaxes them, and still others enjoy classical music, instrumentals, or any kind of vocals. Both of us have our own favorite kinds of music to listen to when stressed, and we've both found that after listening to that favorite music we feel better, more energized, and ready to get back to the tasks at hand.

Laughter

> **Laughter is one of the best stress-relievers there is . . . . Muscles relax and endorphins begin to flow.**

Laughter is one of the best stress-relievers there is—in fact, it's a very close second to exercise. Some people even may rank it first. Laughing gets the whole body and mind working. Muscles relax and endorphins begin to flow. Researchers have found that people in hospitals who watched comedy TV shows or funny movies and laughed out loud recovered faster than those who didn't. So laugh a lot!

Maybe it's a funny movie, a funny TV show, a visit to a comedy club, or just a talk with someone who makes you laugh. Whatever makes you laugh will help. And it even will help those who don't *think* it will help!

Humorist C. W. Metcalf makes a career out of teaching people how to laugh. He uses his suggestions in his own life too. One of the things that helps him relax and laugh is putting on a red clown nose as he drives home from work. "It's hard to take yourself too seriously when you're wearing a clown nose," Metcalf says, "and besides, you see some awfully funny reactions from a lot of people." You don't have to wear a clown nose to laugh. But if you think it could help, give it a try.

- Janice has a collection of what she calls "dumb movies" that help her get through stressful times. "They may be dumb, but they make me laugh," she says, "and I always feel better after laughing out loud." Janice often likes to combine her movie watching with exercise so she can benefit from two stress-reduction techniques at once. "I'm on my treadmill every day," she states, "and when I'm really stressed I walk longer and watch a funny movie at the same time."

Managing Stress Effectively

Movies are just one way to start laughing. Find whatever appeals to your sense of humor. Try it—you'll realize that laughing is one of the best stress relievers there is!

Strategy 2: Talk It Out

Some people find it helpful to talk out their stress with someone else. What do they talk about? They vent. They spout. They show their anger. They get their feelings out in the open. The dynamic appears to be this: Some people simply need to hear themselves say things. When they verbalize their frustration or anger, it becomes easier to deal with it and then to set it aside.

> **Some people simply need to hear themselves say things. When they verbalize their frustration or anger, it becomes easier to deal with it and then to set it aside.**

This someone else can be a friend, spouse, parent, child, neighbor, coworker, pastor, rabbi, or professional counselor. The important thing is having someone to talk with. Talking out your stress doesn't mean that you're looking for agreement or sympathy—just someone who will sit, listen, be genuinely interested in you, and let you talk.

The person doesn't even need to say much other than to let you know he or she is listening and is interested in what you have to say. If this person ever has been where you are now, that's often an added plus. Here's what others have said:

- "My sister is a great listener. I can spout off about all I'm going through and get it out of my system."

- "It's interesting the way it works. Once I hear myself say something, it's out in the open where I can deal with it or walk away from it."

- "Usually just telling my significant other about how stressed I am is all it takes. Then I feel better, and it doesn't bother me as much. I'm ready to get back into it the next day."

If you're a person who is helped by talking out your stress, find someone with whom you can talk. You might even find it helpful to share time: You listen to the other person for 30 minutes, and then the other person listens to you.

Strategy 3: Anticipate Times of Stress

By planning ahead and anticipating times of stress, you often can reduce its impact. Periodically review your calendar (every week or two—whatever works for you). Project yourself into the future, and identify those times coming up that have the potential for being stressful. When you identify a period of possible high stress, plan for it.

● Managing Stress Effectively

First, admit to yourself that you're going to experience some extra stress so it doesn't catch you by surprise. Second, develop a plan to help you reduce as much of the stress as possible. For example, if you're having a high-stress week at work and you also do the cooking at home, ask for help with the chores at home so you'll have extra energy to deal with the stress at work. Or just plan to eat out.

> **When you're in the midst of the high-stress time, stop momentarily to check on how you're doing.**

Third, put your plan into action. When you're in the midst of the high-stress time, stop momentarily to check on how you're doing. Be sure you've made time to do the things that will help you relieve stress—exercising, talking, listening to music—and be sure to get extra sleep. Most people benefit from extra sleep when they're trying to combat stress.

- Steve and Cindy are a dual-career couple, and between them their pace gets rather hectic. One is business manager for a clinic and the other is a floor nurse in ICCU. When they know in advance that things will be hectic, they note it, talk about it, and make a plan to deal with it. But how do they always know in advance?

  They don't! As you're aware, ICCU can explode with work at a moment's notice. The clinic can move from slow to hectic in a few hours. But often they can anticipate times of stress, because of scheduling, planned absences, or extra work because of what week it is. Even when they can't anticipate, once the hectic time hits, they plan on dealing with their stress.

  "The key," Cindy reports, "is that we talk about it and anticipate those times when stress may be high, and then we get ourselves ready for it."

Strategy 4: Reward Yourself

Rewards can help you deal with stress. They make you feel good about getting something done, and, in the midst of a stressful time, they give you something pleasant to look forward to when it's all over.

- A strategy Terri likes is to reward herself for her efforts to reduce stress, and she often use it in conjunction with the strategy on planning for times of stress. When she knows of a stressful time ahead, she plans for it. Then when it's over, she goes out and rewards herself. Maybe it's having a dinner out, buying a new blouse, or doing something else that's enjoyable. A reward can be something as simple as buying gourmet ice cream or leaving work early. Rewards can be almost anything, and they don't have to cost much.

  What's important is that Terri plans ahead and tells herself, "You have a real busy couple of days coming up, with more to do than

Managing Stress Effectively

you have time or energy for. But you'll get it all done, just like you have in the past. Then, when it's all behind you, you can reward yourself with . . ." Fill in the blank.

Strategy 5: Volunteer

> For many people, volunteering is an effective way to manage stress.

For many people, volunteering is an effective way to manage stress. They might volunteer as part of a neighborhood program, or as part of their religious lives, or in some health-related service organization. What's important is that you give of yourself to some agency or program that fits with your own value system.

- "There's something about going and helping people learn how to deal with their newly diagnosed diabetes that is very satisfying," Caesar observes. "It helps me keep my own life in perspective, and I know that I'm doing something important to help others deal with their lives."

Strategy 6: Go for a Drive

Some people reduce stress by going for a drive. As Natalie explains, "It settles me down. Driving for an hour out in the country or even on the highway relaxes me." Lots of folks find relaxation behind the wheel.

It's not so much that they're going anywhere, but simply that they're controlling their car—their machine—while they're driving. Although most of us prefer not to drive in high-traffic areas, some report that congested traffic doesn't bother them when they drive to relieve stress. Here's what others have said:

- "It gives me more to think about as I work my way through traffic, and I find that I have lots of patience."

- "I always have a destination—maybe a park, a nearby river, a favorite shopping center, or a restaurant. When I get there, I spend some time, and then head back. It's a great way to unwind and spend a Saturday afternoon."

Strategy 7: Use Moderation

Once, when we were discussing these stress-reduction strategies with a group of employees whose work unit had just been sold, someone said, "I use the six-pack method of reducing stress." The group laughed. "Yes sir," the employee continued, "I go out and buy a six-pack and by the time it's all gone, I always feel a lot better."

Richard didn't laugh with the others. Why? Because at one time, the "six-pack method" also was his primary way of reducing stress. It took him several months to realize that:

- It was expensive.
- He always had a terrible headache the next morning.
- Others really didn't think he was very pleasant or funny.
- He was using "the six-pack method" more and more often.
- The stress always was still there the next day.

With the help of some understanding friends, he was able to set that particular strategy aside.

A very effective strategy to replace it is simply to use moderation—in just about everything. Use moderation in drinking, in eating, in sleeping, and yes, even in exercise. Too much exercise, especially if you're not already in shape, can create more problems than it solves.

Strategy 8: Use Your Conative Strengths

Remember our earlier discussion of conation and why everyone doesn't react to change the same way? One of the reasons we get stressed in the first place is that we weren't given the chance to use our natural energy in the action area of our strongest conative instincts. When we become stressed, one way to reduce the stress is to do the things that come naturally to us. Using your conative strengths is one of the most effective ways to reduce stress.

> When we become stressed, one way to reduce the stress is to do the things that come naturally to us. Using your conative strengths is one of the most effective ways to reduce stress.

- **Fact Finders**, for example, become stressed when they don't have all the information they feel they need. One way they can reduce their stress is to do some probing, researching, and information gathering, such as reading a book or a magazine, watching a TV documentary, enjoying a mystery, or taking time to read the newspaper without interruption. Many Fact Finders report that the more stress they're under, the more books they read.

  If you think you have a lot of natural Fact Finder instincts and are under stress, use your conative instinct: Do that research you've been meaning to get to, read those reports that have been piling up on your desk, catch up on your professional journals, or just read whatever it is you enjoy reading.

- **Follow Thrus** become stressed when the organizational structure is changed or is in limbo, when they can't see how things all will fit together, or when there's no sense of closure or completion to

Managing Stress Effectively

anything. One way they can reduce their stress is to organize something, like their office, their desk, or a filing cabinet. One person told me he had the best-organized office in the department, as well as the best-organized closet at home. He reviewed his project files and reorganized them to better fit his future needs. At home, he organized his clothes by season and by color within each season, and then by whether they were for work, dress, or casual wear.

If you think you have a good deal of Follow Thru instincts, you deal with stress by organizing your office, your desk, your station, or whatever needs your special talent at keeping things in order. Bring something to completion.

- **Quick Starts** can become stressed during organizational change when the change doesn't occur fast enough or when not enough new things are taking place to utilize their natural energy. When that happens, Quick Starts can energize themselves by starting something new or by coming up with a new way to do something that isn't being done as well as it could be.

Make use of your Quick Start talent. When you're stressed, go to work on a new project, take a look at an old problem to see if you can come up with a new solution, or identify a project that needs your innovative talents.

> **Whatever your conative instincts, you can use them to help reduce stress. To deny these conative strengths, or "to go against the grain" will only add to your frustration.**

- **Implementors** become stressed when there's no physical action, when they fear that the quality of what's being produced is about to be compromised, or when the quality of the tools they need to be productive may be sacrificed. When this happens, Implementors need to do something physical or work with their hands.

If you are an Implementor dealing with stress, build or repair something, work in the yard, wash the car, go for a walk, cross-stitch, lift weights, cook, or do whatever you find enjoyable that uses your Implementor instincts. Implementors can reduce stress by doing something physical.

Whatever your conative instincts, you can use them to help reduce stress. To deny these conative strengths, or "to go against the grain," will only add to your frustration.

Strategy 9: Interact With a Pet

> For many people, pets reduce stress, increase happiness, and add to longevity.

Research has shown that for many people, pets reduce stress, increase happiness, and add to longevity. A dog or cat seems to work best because they're the easiest pets with which to form an emotional bond. They can be petted, handled, touched, cared for, and in return show all kinds of unconditional affection.

Pets are just plain glad to see you, and that's nice to come home to at the end of a hectic day.

- "My retriever, Cher, and I spend hours together," Maury says. "And mornings when I don't want to jog, but need to, Cher is there reminding me it's time to get moving. Yes, I always feel better after my exercise, and Cher always is glad to see me when I get home after the night shift."

Strategy 10: Challenge Your Mind-Set

> Unless an event is life-threatening, it's stressful only if we choose to let it be stressful.

This strategy has to do with *mind-set*—the way you think. Psychologist Albert Ellis pointed out many years ago that unless an event is life-threatening, it's stressful only if we choose to let it be stressful. In other words, it's how we interpret an event that determines our reactions to it—not the event itself.

- Imagine that you've had to work 20 minutes beyond your usual break time for lunch. Being 20 minutes late for lunch is the event. How you interpret that event determines your reaction to it. If you say something like, "Well, I don't like being late because I'm hungry, but it's no big deal," then your reaction will reflect that it's no big deal to you. You'll go ahead and simply be 20 minutes late for lunch.

  On the other hand, if you interpret that event and say to yourself something like, "This is terrible. It shouldn't have happened, and I'm very angry at the imposition," then your reaction will reflect that interpretation. You'll be angry, and because of your anger, you'll probably get indigestion when you finally do eat lunch.

  In both cases, the event is the same, but the reactions are greatly different. What makes the difference is how you interpret the event—your mind-set.

During organizational change, you have the opportunity to challenge your mind-set. Your interpretation of the change will determine your reaction to it. If you say something like, "This is terrible, the worst thing that's ever happened to me, and I'll never get over it," then that's probably what will happen. You probably never *will* get over it. The organizational change will have an impact on you for a long, long time. You'll waste a lot of energy being angry over something that was beyond your control.

Managing Stress Effectively

What *is* within your control, however, is your mind-set. If you choose, you can interpret the event like this: "Gee, this isn't the most fun I've ever had, and I'll be glad when it's all over, but for now I'm going to make the most of it." Then your reaction probably will be to make the most of the organizational change, and you'll likely get your work done and remain someone who others enjoy working with. Yes, you'll probably experience some stress, but not enough to make the job unbearable. And you'll get over it.

Still More Strategies

The above strategies aren't the only ways to relieve stress. There are many others, including:

- Going for a walk—around the block, in a park, or along a river.
- Sitting and watching a sunrise, a sunset, a lake, or the ocean.
- Shopping—whether just looking or buying.
- Reading a good book.
- Watching a movie or a play.
- Participating in a sport—or just being an active spectator or fan.
- Sexual activity—always a great way to relax.
- Working at a hobby—stained glass, cross-stitch, cooking, stamp collecting, genealogy, whatever and wherever your conative strengths take you.
- Reflection, meditation, or prayer.
- Keeping a journal or diary.

> If you're going to make change work for you, you have to deal with stress in positive ways

Remember, stress works on you and gets you down. If you're going to make change work for you, you have to deal with stress in positive ways—and it all begins with the commitment to do something instead of nothing.

● **Managing Stress Effectively**

Action!

Take time to identify the most common ways you reduce stress, and write them below. After you've compiled your list of most-used strategies, see if you can identify any patterns as to which ones you use under which stress conditions.

_____

_____

_____

_____

Now review the list of strategies from this chapter. Select three that you've never used before, but for some reason intrigue you. Write these three strategies below, and indicate when you might try one to see how it works for you.

_____

_____

_____

_____

Stress can be a by-product of organizational change. But that's okay, because stress seems to be, like change itself, a natural phenomena. After all, sometimes it is stress that pushes us into new dimensions and new horizons. What's important for you is that you know how to effectively manage stress. When you can manage any stress that comes as a result of organizational change, you increase your ability to make change work for you.

Chapter Six

Seven Strategies for Making Change Work in Health Care

Once you and your team decide to make change work for you, you need to develop the skills to follow through on that decision. In this chapter, we'll introduce you to seven strategies for making change work in health care. These strategies work! We know, because they've already worked in admitting, in pharmacy, in cath lab, in med-surg, in accounting, in marketing, and in every other department found in a health-care setting.

As you read about each strategy, take time to think it through. Sit back and let the information soak in. Ask yourself:

- **"Am I willing to do something instead of nothing?"**
  Without your commitment to making change work, the strategies have little opportunity to make a difference.

- **"Am I willing to take a calculated risk?"**
  Yes, there's risk involved in using any of these strategies. There's always risk when you deal with change because we can never be 100% certain of what change will bring. But without risk, people would never move away from home, find a job, make a friend, fall in love, or experience many other positive things. Remember, there's also a risk in doing nothing.

- **"When can I put this strategy into action?"**
  Some of the strategies involve mind-set, how a person thinks about change. Other strategies involve specific actions for you to take. It will not be enough for you to just read through this chapter. You must make a commitment to put as many of those strategies that fit your situation into action as soon as possible.

With these points in mind, here are seven strategies for making change work in health care:

1. View change as opportunity.

2. Be someone others enjoy working with.

3. Practice effective stress-management strategies.

> **Without your commitment to making change work, the strategies have little opportunity to make a difference.**

Seven Strategies for Making Change Work in Health Care

4. Build bridges, not fences.
5. Exit if you must.
6. Ask the consultant's question.
7. Know what you do best and where you best fit.

Strategy 1: View Change As Opportunity

Several years ago while Richard was leading a workshop on career change for nurses, a participant came up and said something like this: "Dick, whenever I think of change, I think CEO." That's nice, he responded, waiting for the person to continue.

"Sure," she continued, "CEO—Change Equals Opportunity! If you want to be CEO of your life—you know, the decision maker for how you live—you need to think like a CEO. And CEO can mean Change Equals Opportunity!"

The woman was very insightful. The first strategy for making change work is to challenge yourself to think in terms of change as opportunity. As we've seen, without change, none of us would be where we are today. Change has opened our horizons, has enabled us to grow, has brought us to today. With every change in our lives has come new opportunities.

Change is with us all the time. We can view it as tragic, unwanted, or inconvenient. Or we can be CEOs of our own lives and remind ourselves that Change Equals Opportunity.

Action!
Think back through your own personal and professional history. Identify and briefly describe at least three times that change was really an opportunity.

1. _____
   _____
2. _____
   _____
3. _____
   _____

● Seven Strategies for Making Change Work in Health Care

Strategy 2: Be Someone Others Enjoy Working With

Think of the people with whom you work. What are some of the characteristics of the people you enjoy working with? What is it you like and enjoy about working with them? Is it what they say? what they do? how they smile? whether or not they ever laugh?

Now think of people you don't enjoy working with. What is it you don't like? The words they say? The way they look at someone else?

Now, focus on the characteristics of the people you enjoy working with—and put those qualities into action!

> **Focus on the characteristics of the people you enjoy working with—and put those qualities into action!**

Strategy 2 is that simple. We all know it, but sometimes in the midst of organizational change, we forget that nobody likes to work alongside a someone who conveys a negative attitude through complaining or grouchiness.

■ Shawn always enjoyed her work in the dialysis unit, even though some days were long and very emotional, and got along well with her coworkers. But last year she had to deal with the pressures of consolidating two dialysis units in the city and conflicts with a teenage son. Some days, the stress seemed like more than she could deal with.

"That's when my team pulled me aside, and we talked," Shawn recalls. "They pointed out that I had been uncharacteristically short tempered with a couple of patients earlier in the week and that, frankly, I wasn't any fun to work with anymore. They told me that I'd had a negative response for anything anybody said. If someone said it was nice outside, I'd say, 'Yeah, but the wind's blowing.' If someone told about one of their kids' accomplishments, I'd say, 'Just wait until she grows up.' I never had anything positive to say about anything."

"I hadn't realized I'd been that difficult to work with," Shawn continues. "I decided it was time to do something about it. What's been interesting was that when my attitude at work improved, things improved at home too."

As you deal with change, make a conscious effort to be the type of person others enjoy working with. Project a positive attitude, smile, and remember to say "Please" and "Thank You." Finish your own projects on schedule, show interest in your coworkers, compliment their work, and lend a helping hand when needed.

Seven Strategies for Making Change Work in Health Care

When you're a person others enjoy working with:

- More gets done.
- Work is less stressful.
- Going to work is more satisfying.
- The whole workplace is more enjoyable.
- You know how to make change work for you!

> **Action!**
> List some of the characteristics of the people with whom you enjoy working.
>
> _____
> _____
> _____
> _____
>
> You know what to do with the list.

Strategy 3: Practice Effective Stress-Management Strategies

As we saw in Chapter 5, organizational change of any type often results in stress. If you are experiencing stress as your health-care unit adapts to change, then practice the effective stress-management strategies we discussed earlier. You can also reduce stress levels for yourself, your coworkers, and your patients by:

- Controlling your emotions instead of letting your emotions control you.
- Ignoring rumors.
- Accepting that change is taking place throughout health care as well as in all other kinds of organizations.
- Taking care of yourself physically.
- Not acting out of anger.

Accept that change is taking place throughout health care as well as in all other kinds of organizations.

Seven Strategies for Making Change Work in Health Care

There are many strategies for managing stress. The key is to decide to do something instead of nothing—and then do it.

> **Action!**
> Review your notes from Chapter 5, "Managing Stress Effectively." Identify at least three strategies you can implement this week to help you more effectively manage any stress you may be experiencing:
>
> 1. _____
>
> 2. _____
>
> 3. _____

Strategy 4: Build Bridges, Not Fences

New people are a part of most organizational change. Maybe you have a new president, a new manager, or a new supervisor. Maybe you find yourself working with new people in a new unit or a new team.

As you encounter these new people, strive to build bridges, not fences. Fences block you in, keep you from getting anywhere, and can be a hazard to future activities. Bridges, on the other hand, enable you to get from here to there, particularly when the journey involves some rough terrain.

One of the most significant things you can do to build bridges is to give new people a chance.

One of the most significant things you can do to build bridges is to give new people a chance. This may seem difficult at first. You'll remember from Chapter 2 that when we liked the people with whom we worked before, we tend to set up barriers to liking any new people who enter the scene. To build bridges with new team members, you'll have to overcome this natural tendency. Following these steps can help:

1. Get acquainted. Find extra time (lunches, breaks, breakfasts, after hours) to learn about these people. What have they been doing? How do they enjoy it? What do they think are the problems this new unit will experience? Find out as much as you can about these new people because in the process, you'll probably find you like working with them, just as you enjoyed working with your last group.

2. Learn the agenda. Find out the priorities of this new unit. Find out how the unit prefers to work together. Let team members know

Seven Strategies for Making Change Work in Health Care

the conditions in which you are the most productive as you find out how they are the most productive.

3. Get interested in these new people. After all, you will be spending about a third of each day working with them. You'll all enjoy it more if you have an interest in what these people do and what their lives are like. You'll also be more productive, which leads to even more enjoyment. The more we know about people, the easier it is to like them.

You'll all enjoy your work more if you have an interest in what these people do and what their lives are like.

■ MaryJo had been working in the quality enhancement area for seven years, spending most of her time in the east campus of a multi-campus hospital. Then management decided to merge the quality enhancement work from the three campuses into one unit and reduce the number of people in the combined unit. MaryJo found herself working with people she didn't know, since most of her previous team transferred to other work areas outside the quality arena.

"It was spooky, at first," MaryJo reports, "because there were people I had met once in a while, but we never really worked together. I was the newcomer. But they were wonderful!"

The newly formed unit held a special lunch for MaryJo and two other newcomers. The focus? What people did in their spare time. "I learned that two others had a similar interest in classical music," MaryJo says, "and we instantly had a lot to talk about. The transition suddenly became more enjoyable."

Later in the week the new unit met again to talk about ways to enhance their work—not only the environment in which they worked, but also the quality of the information they provided. "We set a ground rule that everybody's ideas were listened to," MaryJo states, "and that afterward we'd break into smaller task forces to come up with what we thought were the top three suggestions. It worked; people listened to what I had to say, we listened to each other, and we came up with some very good ideas to increase the usefulness of what we provide. In fact, I haven't been this excited about work in a long time!"

Seven Strategies for Making Change Work in Health Care

Action!

List at least three ways in which you can help build bridges and not fences.

1. _____

2. _____

3. _____

Now list when you will put these ideas into action.

1. _____

2. _____

3. _____

Strategy 5: Exit If You Must

Sometimes a change is so drastic, you realize that you just can't adapt to it. You are experiencing too much stress, or you don't agree with the new focus and direction, or you find that some other factor is making you uncomfortable. If you come to the conclusion that you just can't deal with the level of change, the best strategy is to exit.

It doesn't do you, your health-care organization, your family, or anyone else any good if you're in a place you don't want to be. You won't be productive. You won't have a feeling of satisfaction. You won't have good health. Those who have to work with you certainly won't enjoy it.

> If you come to the conclusion that you just can't deal with the level of change, the best strategy is to exit.

Seven Strategies for Making Change Work in Health Care

If your organization has a voluntary severance plan, volunteer for it. If not, then identify what you want your next job to be. Also identify the kind of work environment in which you can be productive and satisfied at the same time. Develop your job-search strategy and make the move as quickly as possible.

- "The change was more than I could take," Carmen explains, "and though I wished them well, I felt the new direction was not one I could be productive in. After a great deal of thought, I decided it was time to move on." Carmen's new executive seemed to sense her hesitancy to continue and asked to meet with her.

    "Carol listened to my concerns," Carmen says, "and agreed with some of them. She briefly explained her position and what she wanted to accomplish. And then she asked for my reactions. I told her where I didn't think I fit in, and then went on and said I'd made the decision to exit. That's when she surprised me," Carmen adds. "She offered me assistance to find a place where I could be fully productive and in sync with the organization's goals. That was great!"

    Carmen took several weeks to identify her best skills and the values that were important to her. Then, with the help of the career management specialist provided by her soon-to-be-former employer, she described the kind of environment in which she preferred to work. After about eight weeks, she was in a new position with a smaller organization who needed someone with her skills and values. "It was a great experience," Carmen states, "and put me in control of my life."

Remember that until you exit you still need to get your work done.

Not every organization helps those who want out. But many do. And we know that more will in the future. Remember, however, that until you exit you still need to get your work done. You may not always feel like it, but it's important that you do. If you don't, it's likely that the word will get around and successfully transitioning into a new position with a new company could become much more difficult.

Strategy 6: Ask the Consultant's Question

Consultants contribute to an organization's efforts by continually asking one question—*What needs doing that isn't being done . . . or could be done better?*—and then coming up with solutions that work.

One of the most effective strategies you can use to make change work in health care is to ask the consultant's question. As you do your own work, constantly look for things that aren't being done that need to get done or could be done better. It might be something as simple as the need to move a wastebasket from one place to another so people won't fall over it. Or it could be more complex, such as implementing a new technology to reduce time and error in dispensing medications.

Seven Strategies for Making Change Work in Health Care

Here are several examples of what others have come up with, just because they took the time to ask the consultant's question:

- When the community hospital added an exercise therapist to their rehab unit, they realized the specialist had extra time. Someone asked, "How can we make use of this person's expertise?" As the department explored ways to share this expertise, they found out that there was no one else in the community performing the same functions. After several meetings with area fitness centers and the local Y, a cooperative program was developed so that the other organizations could have access to and regular use of the specialist. It was the first joint program between the hospital and other community organizations. Someone stopped and asked, "How else can this person's expertise be used in this community?"

- In a major hospital, a programmer designed a computer program to eliminate redundant paperwork. Now when an item is ordered, the system automatically adds it to future inventory, advises accounts payable of future costs, and advises internal users of when the item will be available. Why? Because someone realized that with the power of computers, there had to be a way to enter information once and make it do more than just one thing.

> **What needs doing that isn't being done or could be done better in your organization?**

- When two physician groups merged, they experienced an immediate clash of cultures. Each office was challenged with sharing resources, new policies, and conflicting work environments. It was close to falling apart when the two office managers started asking the employees, "What needs doing that isn't being done?" Responses came quickly! Several task forces were formed with representatives from each of the two offices. The employees soon realized that the focus should be on creating a new culture that more effectively served the patients while enhancing the work environment. Though it took several months, the new culture began to emerge. Both patient satisfaction and employee satisfaction are higher than in either of the two previous offices.

What needs doing that isn't being done or could be done better in your organization?

Once you've identified something that needs doing that isn't being done or could be done better, you need to develop a plan. You may be able to come up with a plan by yourself, or you may need the assistance of other team members who are knowledgeable about the possible action.

Seven Strategies for Making Change Work in Health Care

Develop your plan in as much detail as possible, including what you want to accomplish, why, the resources needed to take the plan into action, and the projected results. Remember, the results need to be significant enough to support the action. For example, a new system to enroll participants doesn't solve much if it costs more than the existing system and does nothing to reduce error or enhance patient or member satisfaction.

As you build your action plan, remember to think in terms of what key decision makers will look for as justification for your idea.

As you build your action plan, remember to think in terms of what key decision makers will look for as justification for your idea. And finally, be ready to respond to objections. If your idea hasn't been done before there will be objections, and you will need to be ready to respond.

When your plan is ready, take it to the right decision maker. Maybe that person is your immediate manager, or maybe it's someone else. But your efforts will be to no avail if you take your plan to someone who will do nothing about it.

Does all of this work? Yes! Is this skill important? Yes!

We believe this skill is so essential that by the year 2005 employers will demand it. Employees will be expected to do their work by proactively looking for ways to enhance customer satisfaction, quality of product or service, or reduce or keep costs in line. In a number of health-care organizations this skill is being taught to employees, and employees are relied upon to use the skill each day to enhance organizational effectiveness.

The health-care field needs people who are looking for ways to do things better, or more efficiently, or with fewer resources. Just ask the consultant's question and make change work for you!

Action!

In the next 24 hours that you work, take along an extra notepad or several 3 x 5 cards that you can easily carry. As you do your work, continually be on the alert for things that need doing that aren't being done or could be done better. As you identify possible actions, jot a few notes to yourself so you won't forget. And then begin to develop your plan.

Seven Strategies for Making Change Work in Health Care

Strategy 7: Know What You Do Best and Where You Best Fit

In the traditional workplace, employees didn't often have much to say about their work assignments. The old workplace paradigm went something like: "I'm your manager, and I'll tell you what I want you to do and how to do it."

Today a new paradigm is emerging in the workplace. The new paradigm goes like this: "You tell me where you best fit in the organization."

This is a big shift. We first began noticing this several years ago as we talked with managers who were increasingly looking to their team members for feedback on how to get things done. We began to notice that some managers were asking their people to tell them what they did best and what they needed in order to be fully productive.

> **Employees who can identify where they best fit within the organization are also extremely satisfied and glad to be with that group.**

What we've learned since is that some entire organizations function like this. Employees are asked to identify where they best fit so they can make the most contribution to the organization. What these organizations have learned is that when employees know themselves and their strengths so well that they can identify where they best fit within the organization, they are also extremely satisfied and glad to be with that group. Job satisfaction is high and so is productivity.

People who can tell their team leader what they do best and where they best fit within the organization will continue to have positions. As health-care organizations change—and all health-care organizations will continue to change in the next decade—these people will be able to step forward and identify where they can make the most contribution within the changed environment. They will be in control of their futures. They will know how to make change work for them.

Here's what you can do to identify what you do best and where you best fit.

Step 1: List Your Responsibilities

Take a piece of paper for each of the positions you've held, beginning with your present position. Make a list of the things you did in each of those jobs, and be sure to include special projects that you were involved in, special teams you were part of, and any special assignments. Make your list as detailed as possible. Spend the most time on those jobs that you really enjoyed and believe you did very well.

68

Seven Strategies for Making Change Work in Health Care

Step 2: Ask "So What?"

For each of the items on your list of things you've done, ask yourself "So what?" You are trying to identify the results of your work, and asking yourself "So what?" is the most helpful way to get at those results. Consider these two examples:

- Tim processes statements in the hospital's credit center. He lists the things he does and begins to ask "So what?" As he ponders the results of his work, he realizes that he has a number of them, which include:

  - Reduced error rate to less than 1 percent.
  - Commended by patients and patient families for being courteous and prompt with information.
  - Designed new input form that reduced data entry time by over 30 percent.
  - Trained new employee in data entry, and assisted him in reducing error rate from 6 percent to less than 2 percent within two weeks.
  - Served on team to evaluate procedures and recommend ways to streamline processing.

- Angie is a supervisor in a cardiac rehab program. As she analyzes all that she does, she realizes that she does much more than just monitoring a patient's progress after PTCA's or bypass surgery. In fact, she's made some significant contributions to health care, which include:

  - Provided rehab services for more than 85 percent of all cardiac patients served by the hospital.
  - Led team in process improvement program and identified 11 ways to reduce costs.
  - Developed volunteer program to assist new rehab customers in becoming familiar with the program.
  - Researched and designed a six-month checkup service after people completed the program.
  - Achieved program completion rate exceeding 90 percent.
  - Commended by cardiac surgeons and physicians for ability to quickly identify potential problems and take appropriate actions.

Why focus on results? Because the results you have achieved are a strong indicator of what you do best. The other indicator is that what you do best is typically what you most enjoy doing. And what you most enjoy doing is typically the kinds of things in which you're the most successful!

The results you have achieved are a strong indicator of what you do best.

Seven Strategies for Making Change Work in Health Care

Step 3: Review Your Results

Review the list of results you identified by asking "So what?" Circle or highlight in some way the things you have most enjoyed, or the things you're the most proud of, or the things you did which you believe made the most contribution. What you are trying to identify are the things you've done that illustrate what you do best. Let's return to the two examples above.

- Tim concluded that what he does best is helping patients resolve questions about their bills. How did he come to this conclusion? "It's what I most enjoy doing," Tim explains. "On the days that I've been able to help our customers find answers to their questions, help them work out a payment plan, or file insurance papers, I leave work feeling that it's been a great day."

- Angie realized that what she did best was to take a standard health-care program and find ways to do it better. "It doesn't have to be broke to fix it," Angie states, "and I really enjoy getting to know a program so well that I can find ways to make it even better. That's what I most enjoy doing, and that's how I can be the most helpful to the hospital."

> **After you've identified the things you most enjoy doing in your work, look for the common themes.**

After you've identified the things you most enjoy doing in your work, look for the common themes. Most people have what we call an *umbrella theme,* something that fits over us, covers us, and defines us. Within that umbrella theme, you can usually find about three major skills areas.

Step 4: Describe Your Accomplishments

Find the right words to describe what you do best.

- Tim decides that his overall theme is his ability to solve financially related problems. As he continues to review and reflect on what he does best, he concludes that his three best skills within this theme are:

    - Working directly with patients to resolve financial concerns.
    - Being a coach and mentor to new employees to assist them in learning how to deal with customers' financial concerns.
    - Designing new procedures to enhance customer satisfaction.

    Now Tim is ready to talk with others about what he does best and where he best fits within the health-care organization.

Seven Strategies for Making Change Work in Health Care

- Angie decides that her umbrella theme is that of helping people take control of their health. As she continues to think about what she does best, she begins to realize that what she does best includes:

    - Helping people understand their health situation without being alarmed.
    - Showing hesitant people how to set up a health-management plan which they can easily follow.
    - Designing learning programs to help people recover from major interventions.

    She realized that what she did best was pretty much what she was already doing.

Step 5: Talk with Others

As you identify your umbrella theme and your three major skills or strengths, share that information with others. Get their reactions. Listen to what they have to say about what they have observed of you and your work. Others often have good additional insight into your major strengths. Sometimes we are so close to ourselves, we need someone else to help us step outside ourselves and examine our strengths.

Finally, be ready to talk with others about where you best fit and where you can make the most contribution.

Others often have good additional insight into your major strengths.

Action!

Follow the five steps listed in this chapter to identify what you do best. To help you carry out this activity, write in the space below the date by which time you want to have this strategy completed:

I will be able to talk with others in detail about where I best fit within the organization by _____.

Chapter Seven

Dealing with Downsizings

The numerous changes taking place in health care today have led to a number of reorganizations and downsizings. There can be a variety of reasons for downsizings: Hospitals merge to cut overhead, more outpatient or short-term stay procedures reduce the need for hospital beds, and new procedures and technologies reduce the time even critically ill patients stay in the hospital.

For people who went into a profession to help people, downsizings are not fun. People lose jobs, and personal values often come in conflict with reality. But you don't have to just sit back and watch a downsizing happen. There are a number of things you can do that will make a difference. In other words, you can be part of the solution rather than being part of any problem. If you decide to make change work for you, you'll find that you're a good deal more satisfied with your job, and your coworkers will be grateful for your positive attitude.

> You don't have to just sit back and watch a downsizing happen. There are a number of things you can do that will make a difference.

Taking Action to Stay in Control

What do you do if your health-care organization downsizes? Here are nine actions you can take to deal successfully with downsizing.

Action #1: Keep a Positive Attitude

As we saw in Chapter 6, there's nothing more unpleasant to deal with every day than someone with a sour, negative attitude who only talks about the bad things taking place. That kind of a dark mood can quickly spread over the others. However, the reverse is also true. There's nothing more helpful than a person with a positive attitude who is cheerful, easy to work with, and pleasant to be around. One of the most helpful things you can do for your friends in the work unit is to remain positive—to look for new opportunities, new visions, new goals.

Action #2: Be a Friend

You may have several good friends who exit as part of the downsizing. One action you can take is to remain their friend. Just because they leave doesn't mean you can't continue to do things together or enjoy each other's company. Besides, they will probably want to know what is happening within the health-care organization and who is doing what.

Dealing with Downsizings

Being a friend can include sharing information (like the material presented later in this chapter on the Deems Job Loss Reaction Cycle™), listening when the person needs to vent, and continuing to include the person in social activities.

Action #3: Ask for Help if You Need It

Those left after a downsizing often experience a variety of emotions, from anger to sadness to guilt at having a job when others have lost theirs. If you find that you are having difficulty dealing with your emotions, ask for help. Many communities have special centers to help people deal with job loss, and those centers should have resource persons available to help people who remain after a downsizing.

> If you find that you are having difficulty dealing with your emotions, ask for help.

If your entire work unit finds that it is having trouble dealing with the downsizing, ask your unit manager for some help from the organization. Don't be embarrassed to ask for help. It shows a sense of maturity, self-awareness, and the commitment to make change work for you.

Action #4: Be Supportive of New People

As we observed in Chapter 6, there are almost always some personnel changes in any downsizing. You may find yourself with a new team leader, a new department manager, or a new division executive. You may even find yourself with new people in your work unit.

Give these new people a chance. Listen to what they have to say. Help them get acquainted with your work team's routines and procedures. Help them get acquainted with the people in your work group and in other units with whom you may interact. Everyone involved will appreciate the positive, upbeat approach.

Action #5: Remind Yourself That Managers Are Human Too

Decision makers are not all mean monsters—even if they appear that way sometimes. They are human too. They make mistakes. They don't like doing things that negatively effect other people's lives. They would rather build than take apart. So give them a break.

Treat decision makers as you want to be treated. If you enjoy positive attitudes, smiles, and greetings in the hallways, treat the decision makers the same way. Acknowledge that maybe they're under stress too. Just remember to treat them with the respect and kindness that you like to be treated.

Dealing with Downsizings

Action #6: Do Your Job

The stress is high on everyone during a downsizing, and there's a tendency for productivity and quality to decline. However, a drop in productivity or quality only adds to the stress. You'll find change goes easier for you and your coworkers if you keep up your energy and get your job done on schedule and up to quality expectations. If you don't, you'll be forcing your coworkers to take up the slack.

> You'll find change goes easier for you and your coworkers if you keep up your energy and get your job done on schedule and up to quality expectations.

■ Sonja didn't enjoy seeing some of her friends leave the hospital because of the downsizing. But new technology made some positions redundant. It was only a few weeks after the downsizing that Sonja's coworkers began to notice the extra hours she was putting into her job. "She always stuck around and made sure everything got done," her supervisor says. "And then we realized—Sonja was doing her job and making sure that everything else that was supposed to be done on the shift got done. She kept us all going during a time of high stress."

Be sure and do your job so Sonja doesn't have do yours as well as hers.

Action #7: Make a Commitment

Decide that you're going to make change work for you, and encourage others to make the same kind of commitment. Once you decide to make change work, you'll find that surviving a downsizing is much easier. You'll be able to acknowledge that sometimes it takes extra energy, but your work unit wants to be part of the solution and not part of the problem.

Action #8: Remind Yourself of What Things Were Like Before Downsizing

In the midst of organizational change, those who remain often forget the many things they really didn't like before downsizing took place. So stop and remind yourself what it was like before downsizing. After all, you may find that you like things a whole lot better now than before.

Action #9: Take Time to Understand the Job Loss Reaction Cycle

There is a normal reaction cycle experienced by those who go through job loss. Even employees who remain after a downsizing go through the cycle. When you understand the cycle, and accept the reactions as normal, you are making change work for you.

Dealing with Downsizings

Following the Deems Job Loss Reaction Cycle™

> **Employees who remain after a downsizing go through a reaction pattern in the same way as those whose jobs have been eliminated.**

Employees who remain after a downsizing go through a reaction pattern in the same way as those whose jobs have been eliminated. The only difference is the level of intensity. People who lose their jobs typically react to job loss with greater intensity than those who remain and who then watch their friends and coworkers exit.

This cycle was first identified in the early 1980s as Richard's work turned from helping people deal with terminal illness or the death of a loved one to assisting those who had gone through job loss. As his work shifted, he realized that there were some major differences in the reaction patterns.

As Richard's research base expanded, he identified a separate and distinct reaction cycle for losing one's job, as illustrated in Figure 2. In the years since, he has observed that people don't go through this Job Loss Reaction Cycle in a neat, linear, sequential way. Instead, as the arrows indicate, it's an up and down process. People can go through the cycle several times in one day, or they can settle in one stage and get stuck for awhile. Ultimately, most people reach Acceptance and Affirmation and stay there.

```
           Frustration              Fear
              Shock and Disbelief
              Anger and Resentment
              Denial and Bargaining
              Self-Doubt and Put-Downs
              Withdrawal and Depression
              Acceptance and Affirmation

                Physical Reactions
```

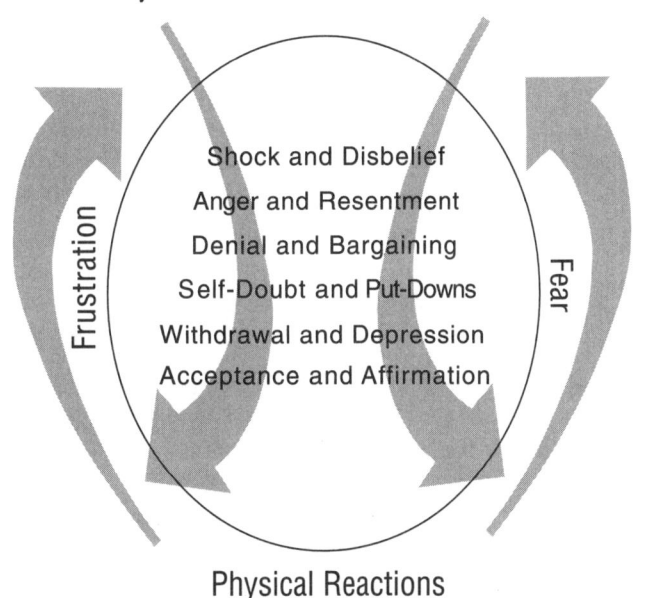

Figure 2—Deems Job Loss Reaction Cycle™

As Figure 2 illustrates, employees who remain after a downsizing also go through this cycle in an atmosphere of *fear, frustration,* and *physical reactions.* There is the fear of further layoffs, or that salaries will get reduced, or . . . (people tend to fill in their own blanks). There is also lots of frustration as survivors have to pick up the work previously done by those who left and deal with the organizational changes that are part of any downsizing.

Dealing with Downsizings

There are also physical reactions, and it is common for work units who continue after a downsizing to experience an increase in colds and flu-like symptoms. For some, there are even more complicated physical reactions, such as ulcers and colitis, and a few may find that some kind of medication is needed to help them deal with the stress.

People who survive a downsizing go through six stages.

Within this environment, people who remain after a downsizing go through six stages:

- **Stage 1: Shock/Disbelief**
  The first immediate reaction is shock and disbelief. Even though there may have been rumors about the downsizing, people still aren't prepared. For most employees, this stage lasts only a few minutes or a few hours.

- **Stage 2: Anger/Resentment**
  Anger and resentment quickly follow. Maybe the anger is directed toward the manager who made the announcement, or to key decision makers, or even the company in general. The anger is caused by many reactions: anger that jobs have to be eliminated, anger over who is and who is not exiting, anger over the need for organizational change, and on and on.

  Over the years, we have seen that is that if this anger isn't dealt with and set aside, it can consume people. Work units who remain must be certain that they have worked through their anger and put it into perspective, or the anger could keep them from doing what's in their own best interests.

- **Step 3: Denial/Bargaining**
  Remaining work units have a tendency to engage in denial and bargaining after a downsizing has been announced. Sometimes they try to fool themselves and deny the reality of the downsizing. "They'll change their minds," is often heard, along with, "Just wait, they'll see how those folks are needed and call them back." Since most downsizings take place only after decision makers have considered many alternatives, the chances of a callback are typically slim to none.

  Bargaining is often very subtle. Productivity often increases after an announcement of a downsizing. It's as if people say to themselves, "Maybe if we work harder, they'll see how much all of us are needed."

- **Stage 4: Self-Doubt/Put-Downs**
  Work units often feel that they are the specific reason for the downsizing. "If only . . ." is often heard, sometimes spoken out loud, and sometimes unspoken. At this point, self-confidence

Dealing with Downsizings

wavers, and employees wonder if they have what it takes to be successful in today's competitive marketplace. What is needed to counteract this dynamic is a reminder of all that they have accomplished. Individual employees need to be reminded of their contributions.

◆ **Stage 5: Withdrawal/Depression**
At some point, individual work units withdraw from others, particularly from management. Employees will seem quiet, almost sullen. Sometimes this withdrawal and depression is a result of feeling guilty over being the remaining ones, those who still have a job.

This stage is similar to the Anger stage. If it's not dealt with and things aren't put into perspective, then it can consume people. Any reactions of guilt over still having a job needs to be dealt with, and feelings of depression need to be confronted. Sometimes entire work units can benefit from meeting with community specialists.

◆ **Stage 6: Acceptance and Affirmation**
This is the goal. This is where work units can say something like

■ Sure didn't enjoy this . . . would have been easier if it hadn't happened . . . but it has, and we're dealing with it. We accept the reality of the situation and know that there is lots of change taking place, and we affirm that we have skills and much to contribute now and in the future.

> **A work unit has reached Acceptance and Affirmation when members can talk about the downsizing and realistically assess the results.**

A work unit has reached Acceptance and Affirmation when members can:

◆ Talk about the downsizing and realistically assess the results.

◆ Accept their own reactions to the job loss experienced by others.

◆ Affirm that they have skills and strengths.

◆ Accept the changing workplace and the need for continued change.

◆ Affirm that they know how, or will find out how, to remain productive in the changing workplace.

◆ Affirm that they make contributions.

Sometimes it just takes time for people to reach, and stay, in Acceptance and Affirmation. Over the years we've learned that:

◆ People who remain after a downsizing go through this cycle just like those who exit, but usually not to the same extent.

Dealing with Downsizings

- It is an up-and-down cycle, and people go back and forth between stages, often like a yo-yo.

- People can be in Acceptance and Affirmation and then suddenly find themselves back in Anger or some other stage for a while before returning to Acceptance.

- Since this is a normal reaction, there isn't anything wrong with people who go through this cycle—they are normal.

If your work unit is going through a downsizing, then you have already begun to go through the cycle. Now that you understand what happens to people who go through job loss and what happens to people who remain with jobs, you can more effectively make change work for you!

Action!

If you've gone through a recent downsizing, discuss this reaction cycle with other team members. Ask if they've also experienced the same reactions. Ask what others have done to help move through the cycle to Acceptance and Affirmation. Ask others what Acceptance and Affirmation means to them. Be ready to share your own reactions. After you've talked with several others who've gone through a downsizing, take time to reflect and write your thoughts in the space below.

_____

_____

_____

_____

_____

_____

• **Developing a Plan for Action**

Chapter *Eight*

Developing a Plan for Action

> The only way you make change work for yourself and for your health-care organization is to develop a plan for using the concepts and strategies that you've learned.

This is a book designed for action. It is not enough to just read the words—you need to do something about them. Take control of your own situation. Commit to do something instead of nothing. The only way you make change work for yourself and for your health-care organization is to develop a plan for using the concepts and strategies that you've learned.

This final chapter is designed so you can:

- Stop and reflect on what you've learned.

- Determine if there are any topics you want to revisit now or in the future to extend your depth of understanding.

- Describe how you want to put the information into action through your Plan for Action.

If you're ready to do more than just talk about making change work for you, read on.

Here are summaries of the key points for each chapter, with an opportunity to identify topics for further reading. Once you've reviewed your learning and indicated areas for further study, you're ready to develop your own Plan for Action. Since we already know that everyone doesn't react to change the same way, it only follows that everyone isn't going to strategize the same way, either.

Identify Your Questions

Making Change Work for You in Health Care begins with a discussion of the changes taking place in health care today. As you're aware, there are many. The shift of responsibility is moving from the health-care provider to the health-care consumer. Technology and new treatment procedures are reducing the time necessary for hospitalization and in-patient care. Hospitals and clinics are continually looking for ways to reduce costs while maintaining patient satisfaction. Managed care has produced many changes and will continue to do so.

Developing a Plan for Action

> **?** Do you still have questions about changes in health care? If so, write them in the space below and reread Chapter 1, looking for your specific answers.
>
> _____
> _____
> _____
> _____

Change is something we experience constantly since birth, and we know a lot about change. We know that self-chosen change is the easiest. We know that we are what we are because of change. We know that the whole workplace, not just the health-care field, is going through considerable change. We know that change is constant. This book is all about presenting new skills for you to become an expert at making change work.

> **?** Do you have questions about the role change plays in life and what we already know about change? If so, reread Chapter 2 after you've identified your questions in the space below.
>
> _____
> _____
> _____
> _____

Everyone doesn't react to change in the same way. The concept of *conation* as developed by management specialist Kathy Kolbe provides many answers to why people differ in their reaction to change. Some people seem to ask "Why?" while others say "Yeah, but . . ." "Why not?" or "Show me." When coworkers understand the conative strengths of each other, they are better equipped to successfully deal with organizational change.

● Developing a Plan for Action

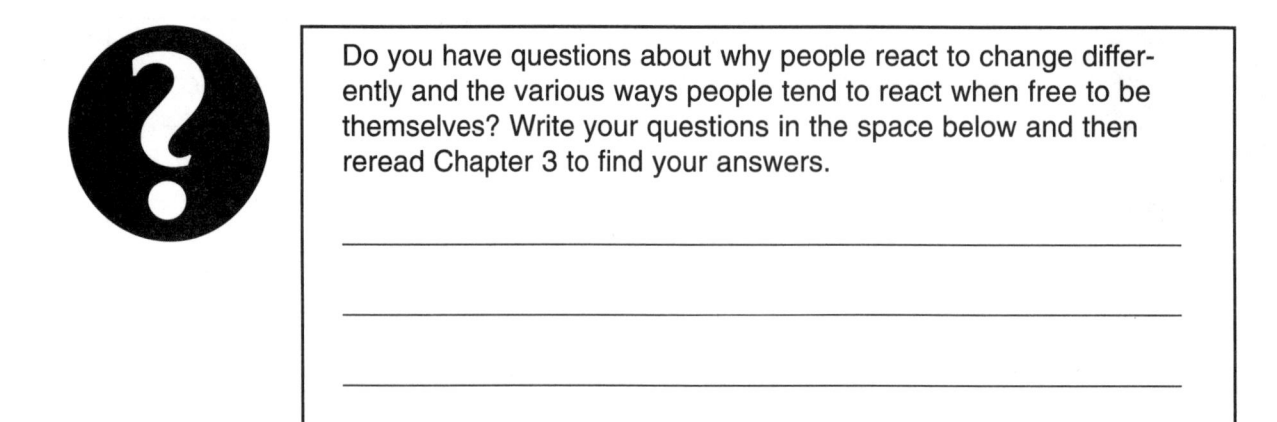

> **?** Do you have questions about why people react to change differently and the various ways people tend to react when free to be themselves? Write your questions in the space below and then reread Chapter 3 to find your answers.
>
> _____
> _____
> _____
> _____

When work units understand that work teams respond to change in predictable patterns, they can identify and describe how they *prefer* their team react to future change. Once they identify the ideal, they can learn the skills so preference becomes reality.

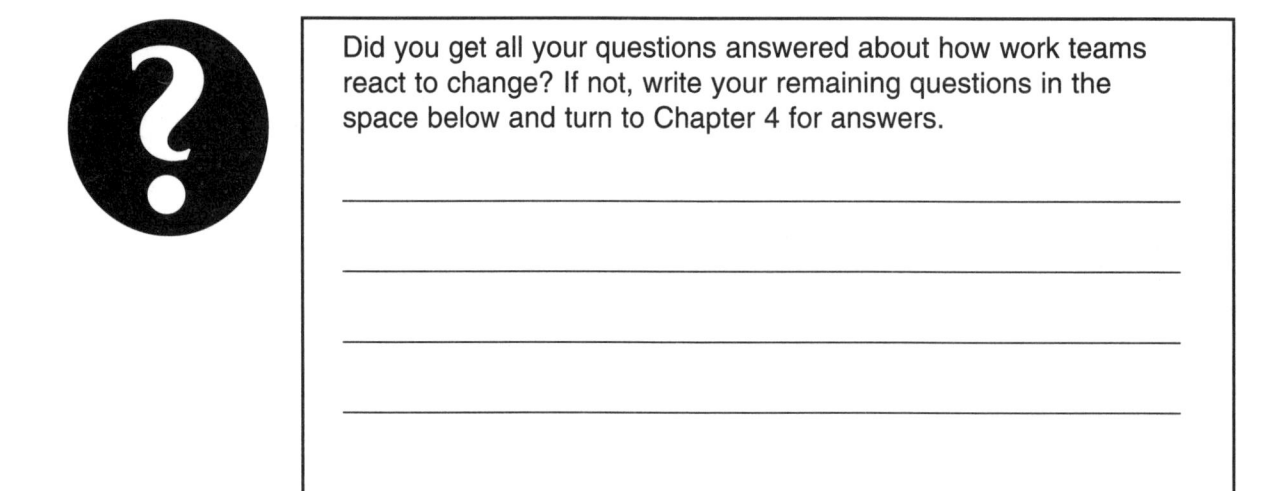

> **?** Did you get all your questions answered about how work teams react to change? If not, write your remaining questions in the space below and turn to Chapter 4 for answers.
>
> _____
> _____
> _____
> _____

Stress seems to be a part of organizational change for just about everybody at one time or another. There are many strategies people can use to become effective managers of stress, such as using endorphins, volunteering, or talking it out.

Developing a Plan for Action

> **?** Chapter 5 can answer any questions you might have about how to be an effective manager of stress. Write your questions below.
>
> _____
> _____
> _____
> _____

When you understand the change taking place in health care, the role change plays in life, why everybody doesn't react to change the same way, how work units react to change, and how to manage stress, you're ready to put strategies to make change work into action! Some strategies deal with mind-set, such as looking at change as an opportunity. Some strategies take more time, like looking for what needs doing that isn't being done or could be done better—and then doing something about it. The main thing is that you use these strategies—you put them into action!

> **?** Are there strategies you want to try that you haven't tried already? Do you need to review a new strategy before putting it into action? Do you have questions about strategies to make change work? Write them below and revisit Chapter 6.
>
> _____
> _____
> _____
> _____

Downsizings are a part of health care, just as they are a part of every other workplace. Will they continue? Probably, in some form or to some extent. Are they fun? Not necessarily. But you can learn how to deal with downsizings.

Developing a Plan for Action

> If you have questions about what to do if you remain with an organization after downsizing, write your questions in the space below and reread Chapter 7.
>
> _____
> _____
> _____
> _____

Questions? Review the material again. Talk with others about their reactions to the material and information. The more sure you are of the information, the easier it will be to develop your Plan for Action and turn those plans into reality.

Develop Strategies for Turning Plans into Reality

If everyone doesn't react to change the same way, then everyone doesn't develop a Plan for Action the same way, either. Some will naturally want more detail than others. Others may even resist putting something down on paper. And some may have great intentions, but never seem to put plans into action.

By now you know, however, that you can't become an expert at making change work unless you put strategies into action. Here is a report of how one work team described their plans for putting ideas into action.

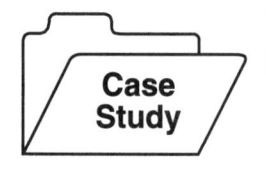

Case Study: Creating a Plan for Action

■ The team had completed a learning program on dealing with change and now, three days later, they meet to talk about how each person is going to use the information and how the group can, together, make change work. Each of the seven team members will be sharing what they had written as their Plan for Action at the end of the workshop.

"What I wrote down was that I'd put the information into action," Jerry began. He paused for a moment, waiting for a reaction. "Three days ago that seemed like all I needed," he added, and the group laughed. Jerry was always coming up with ideas and great intentions. "I'm really serious about this, though."

Developing a Plan for Action

"Maybe you need us to help you get some detail," said Mindy. "So let's get at it."

Mindy asked Jerry to describe three things from the workshop that now, several days later, were important to him. She wrote down on a flip chart what he reported: acknowledging that we are what we are because of change, managing stress, and giving new people a chance.

The group smiled as Jerry talked about giving new people a chance, because his new role put him in daily contact with another team comprised of people from a different building. He had complained several times about "how difficult those new people were to work with." Interestingly, the other group's leader had called and asked how they could work more effectively with Jerry. "He's just not always easy to work with," the new team had reported.

"One of the things that Jerry said really interests me too," Mindy said. "I'd like to explore the concept that we are what we are because of change. As you know, I've gone through some major change myself, what with my dad's sudden death and discovering I was expecting my third child." The discussion continued as both Mindy and Jerry shared additional information about some life and workplace changes that had an impact on them.

"Maybe taking some quiet time to just sit and think and make a list of some of the changes I've dealt with in the last 10 years would help," Jerry said. Jerry continued by describing what made sense to him: making a list of changes, reflecting on each, and writing down the impact each of those changes had on him.

The group applauded Jerry's idea, and Mindy said she thought she'd try something similar too. Then Sandie spoke up. "When are you going to get it done, you two off-the-wall types?" she asked. "Remember, you need challenges, deadlines, a timeline—and the rest of us will be waiting to hear that you finished it too."

Developing a Plan for Action

Mindy laughed and said she wanted it to get it done by the end of the third week. Jerry agreed that a similar timeline would work for him too. Both wrote down their objectives, in specific terms, like this:

Objective	Completed By
1. Make a list of the changes I've experienced in the past 10 years.	2 weeks from today
2. Review each item and identify the impact the change has had on me, focusing more on the positive than the negative.	3 weeks from today

"I think we just realized something about how important it is to be specific about what we want to get accomplished and then set a date when we're supposed to have it done," Catherine said. The group agreed. It doesn't do much good to talk about generalities. Specifics are important when designing a Plan for Action.

"My turn," Brian interjected. "Jerry and I have a similar objective—managing stress. I know guys aren't supposed to get stressed," Brian added, and the others groaned. "But it's been getting to me. Administration says one thing one day and comes back and says something else the next day. It's too much. I want to reduce my stress too."

Brian flipped to a page with lots of notes on it. He described how part of his Plan for Action was to become a more effective manager of stress. He had reviewed his notes and identified five new stress strategies that intrigued him, including some kind of physical fitness program. Then, for each of those five strategies, he listed when he wanted to try each one.

"I've just had another idea," Brian stated. "Listening to us talk about Jerry and Mindy's plans gave me the idea that maybe it would help if I could find other people on the team who had used any of these five stress strategies." Brian read his list and waited.

Barb had begun a new physical fitness program six months earlier, and Scott had signed up as a volunteer at the diabetes center. "If it's all right with you, I'd like to interview you two to see what I can learn about using these strategies," said Brian. "I can do that and still try each strategy by my target date. My plan will work." The others cheered and turned toward Sandie.

Developing a Plan for Action

"Why look at me?" she asked. "I'm still thinking about it." There were some snickers, and Barb reminded Sandie that she often took a lot of time to think about something before she was ready to commit to action. "Okay," Sandie retorted, "this is what I'm thinking about. I'm fascinated by the *consultant's question* strategy, and I'd really like to try it. Part of my Plan for Action is to come up with at least one new procedure to get something done that isn't getting done or could be done better within three months."

Sandie described how she had started to keep a daily journal. In the three days since the workshop, she had identified several things that weren't getting done or could be done better. When she identified something, she quickly made some notes in a small pocket notebook, and at the end of the day she would review any items and write her ideas or observations in a larger notebook. "I've only been doing this for three days," she reminded the others, "but already I've identified five things that could be enhanced."

Sandie shared the rest of her plan, which looked like this:

1. Keep a daily list of things that aren't getting done or could be done better.

2. Review each list and add notes and information for those items which have the greatest interest for me.

3. Research the topic, either at library or by asking others about their reactions and ideas.

4. For the item of greatest interest after three weeks, begin to develop a plan. Ask others on the team for their ideas.

5. Bring in others who can help develop a plan.

6. Develop the plan and share it with the team for their final feedback and support.

7. Present the plan to the person who can decide to do something about it.

● Developing a Plan for Action

Scott was next. "I've used this strategy before," he began "and it helps me keep on target. I want to explore several of the strategies about making change work, so I wrote myself a letter. In the letter, I outlined what I wanted to accomplish by a certain date, and then I asked my cousin to mail the letter so I'd get it two days before my target date."

Scott continued by describing how he had written three letters, one for each of his main objectives. Each was to be mailed to arrive several days prior to his deadline for reaching the objective. "That will give me time to refine and get it accomplished according to my time schedule," Scott added. "It works for me."

Barb had been rather quiet until Sandie reminded her she hadn't reported yet. Barb reached into her notebook and pulled out several pages. "I've taken a different approach," Barb explained. "It's called a *futures invention process*. Basically it asks me to identify what I want to get accomplished, jump into the future to the time I want to have that objective accomplished, break the time into segments from the future point back to the present, and then identify what I have to get accomplished in each time segment in order to get to my objective on schedule."

Barb explained how she had used the futures invention process:

- First, she identified her objective in specific terms and the date by which she wanted to reach that objective. Barb's objective was to reorganize the admissions process, and she wanted to have a plan completed and ready to implement in three months.

- Second, she divided the time from when she wanted to have the reorganization plan completed back to the present into segments. "Month-by-month time segments made the most sense to me," Barb said.

- Third, Barb began at the month segment in which she wanted to have her objective completed. "I began by writing down all the things I would need to do during that time in order to reach my objective on schedule," she said. Then she took the next time segment and asked, "What do I need to do in this time segment in order for me to do those things in the next time segment so I can reach my objective on schedule?"

Developing a Plan for Action

"I thought some of you might be interested in this kind of planning," Barb said, "so I prepared a one-page summary of what I did. Remember," she cautioned, "this doesn't have all the details, but there's enough so you get the idea about ways you can use the futures invention process." Her page looked like this:

Objective: Develop a detailed plan to reorganize the admissions process and department by October 1 (three months into the future).

Activities for Time Segment 3—September
- Final copy typed and ready for distribution
- Review and approval by administration
- Review and refinements (changes) by department task force

Activities for Time Segment 2—August
- First draft of plan prepared for continued review and discussion
- Review task force recommendations
- Review recommendations from focus groups
- Finish focus-group meetings

Activities for Time Segment 1—July
- Identify participants for five focus groups
- Begin conducting focus groups
- Review customer satisfaction reports for the past two years
- Select task force members to assist in developing the plan

Barb picked up a copy of her sample page. "What I didn't include here," she added, "are the dates by which I want to get each of those activities completed. When I've done that, I'll have my entire plan developed, and I'll know what I have to get accomplished each week in order to get to my objective on schedule. No last-minute rushes or late hours trying to play catch-up."

Listening to each other's plans energized the group, and though the day was almost over, the team wasn't ready to wrap up. "We have to put these plans into action," Mindy reminded the group, "or it's a wasted effort."

"Even though we took different strategies, our plans all share two essential features," Sandie observed. "Each plan has an objective and a specific date when we want to reach that objective." Discussion continued as the group agreed that without a clear, specific objective,

● Developing a Plan for Action

there was no plan. There was also no plan if a target date was missing. Sandie reminded them that the objective had to be in measurable and behavioral terms in order to have meaning. "You can measure understanding," she reminded the group, "but only when you think in terms of whether you can describe something, or discuss it, or list the details about it." The team also agreed that without a firm date by which a person wants to reach an objective, there is no movement for action.

Jerry grabbed a marker and headed for the white board. "Even though we plan differently, we have these three common guidelines," he reminded the group. He began writing:

Guidelines for Designing a Plan for Action

1. Describe your objective, what you want to accomplish, in specific and behavioral terms.

2. Identify the date by which you want to reach the objective. Be sure the target date is realistic and achievable.

3. List out your action steps, what it takes to get from "here," where you are now, to "there," where you want to be, on schedule.

The group applauded Jerry's summary. "Now," Barb stated, "it's time to put talk into action!"

Create Your Plan for Action

Turning talk into action and ideas into realities—that's what your Plan for Action is. Develop a realistic and workable plan to make change work for you. Putting your ideas into a Plan for Action follows the three guidelines the team identified. Here's how you can do it.

1. State your objective. Make it clear, specific, and use measurable and behavioral terms. Reread your objective to be sure it is realistic and attainable.

   Write your objective below:

   _____

Developing a Plan for Action

2. Establish the target date by which time you want to have reached your objective. Reread your target date to be certain it is realistic and attainable.

   Write your target date below:

   _____

3. Identify your strategies to reach your objective on schedule. As you read earlier, there are many strategies a person can use to attain an objective on schedule. Select the style that works best for you. Remember, however, that your strategies must be realistic and in enough detail so you know what you have to do in order to reach your objective on schedule.

   Identify your strategies below:

   _____

   _____

   _____

There is yet one more action you can take to help you reach your objective on schedule. Take the time to identify things you can do to make certain you work your plan. For some people, just writing their Plan for Action on paper and setting it aside is enough. For others it isn't. Here are seven actions you can take to remind yourself to continue working your plan.

- Set out a reminder note on your desk or someplace where you'll see it often. The reminder note can read "How are you coming on your Plan for Action?" or whatever it is that will remind you to stick with your plan.

- Write periodic reminder notes in your calendar or planner. Space them at intervals so you'll remember to keep working your plan.

- Make a list of the obstacles you might encounter which might block reaching your objective on schedule. For each potential obstacle, identify one action you can take to neutralize that obstacle.

- Set a scheduled time at the end of each day, or several days, or week, to evaluate your progress toward reaching your objective on schedule.

Developing a Plan for Action

- Ask others to regularly ask you for a progress report. Ask them to make it fun—but to keep you to your schedule.

- Build in rewards. When you reach certain progress points, give yourself a reward: dinner out, an extra game of golf, a new CD, or whatever it is that serves as a reward for you.

- Remain open to serendipity. Serendipity is when, as you are on the road to some established objective, something of equal or greater value shows up. Be open to it. Be ready for it. Be flexible. And be open to changing your objective or plans if it makes sense!

Action!

In the space below describe the actions you can take to help you bring your Plan for Action into reality:

_____
_____
_____
_____
_____
_____

Congratulations! By studying this book, completing the interactive exercises, assessing where you might need to spend some extra time, and developing your Plan for Action, you're ready to make change work for you. You know that change is a universal human experience. Everyone goes through it. And you know that change in the workplace will continue.

None of us knows exactly what a change will involve, but we know there is more change ahead for each of us. We can fight it, or we can make it work for us. As Ken Blanchard stated, "If you learn to accept change, communicate about it, and tackle your goals, you can find that change will be a wonderful opportunity to fulfill your dreams and your ambitions."

Make change work for you in health care!

Developing a Plan for Action

> **Action!**
>
> What is one way you will use the information from this book in the next 24 hours? Write it in the space below:
>
> _____
>
> _____
>
> _____
>
> _____

Great! Congratulations! Pat yourself on your back! Our experience has been that if you don't use the information from this book in some way in the next 24 hours it may be weeks or months before you return to it. That's inaction, not action. Be good to yourself—put the ability to make change work for you in health care into action each and every day!